ESSENTIAL EMOTIONS

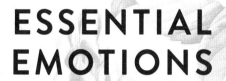

YOUR GUIDE TO
PROCESS, RELEASE,
AND LIVE FREE

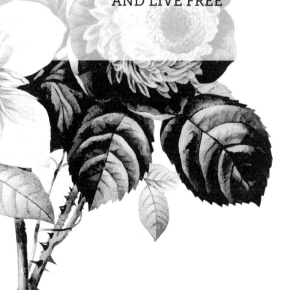

Essential Emotions
YOUR GUIDE TO PROCESS, RELEASE, AND LIVE FREE
9th Edition

ISBN 978-1-7327565-9-5
Printed in the USA
PUBLISHED BY:
Essential Emotions
5513 W. 11000 N. Ste 525
Highland, Utah 84003
www.essentialemotions.com

Thank you to the original Enlighten authors for bringing this work together and for sharing a vision of how these plants can serve to create emotional healing.

We invite you to reference the solutions you find here as you engage the essential oils as powerful tools on your journey to wholeness. Then use the guides to process the emotions, release them, and live in more freedom each day. Thank you in advance for receiving and passing on this life-changing message!

NOTICE TO READERS

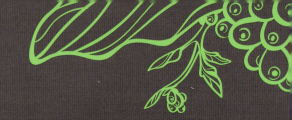

THE MEDICAL SCHOOL OF THE FUTURE WILL NOT PARTICULARLY INTEREST ITSELF IN THE ULTIMATE RESULTS AND PRODUCTS OF DISEASE, NOR WILL IT PAY SO MUCH ATTENTION TO ACTUAL PHYSICAL LESIONS, OR ADMINISTER DRUGS AND CHEMICALS MERELY FOR THE SAKE OF PALLIATING OUR SYMPTOMS, BUT

knowing the true cause

OF SICKNESS AND AWARE THAT THE OBVIOUS PHYSICAL RESULTS ARE MERELY SECONDARY, IT WILL CONCENTRATE ITS EFFORTS UPON BRINGING ABOUT THAT

HARMONY BETWEEN

BODY, MIND & SOUL

WHICH RESULTS IN THE RELIEF AND CURE OF DISEASE.

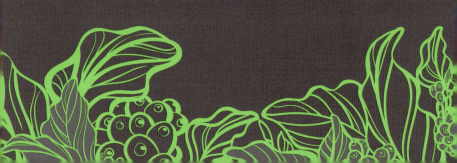

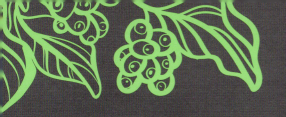

AMONGST THE TYPES OF REMEDIES THAT WILL BE
USED WILL BE THOSE OBTAINED FROM THE MOST

beautiful plants & herbs

TO BE FOUND IN THE

PHARMACY OF NATURE

SUCH AS HAVE BEEN

divinely enriched

WITH

HEALING POWERS

FOR THE MIND AND BODY OF MAN.

– DR. EDWARD BACH –

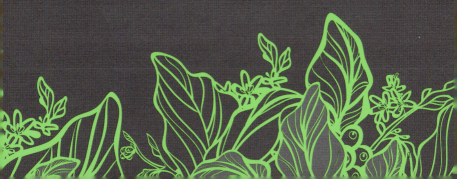

TABLE OF CONTENTS

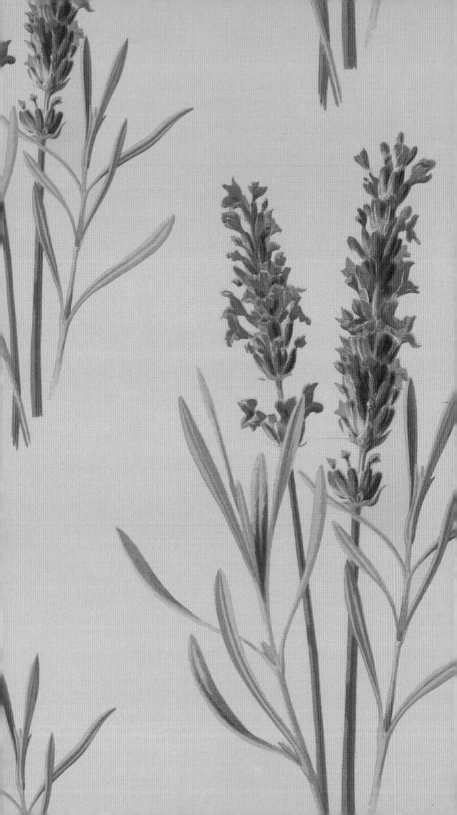

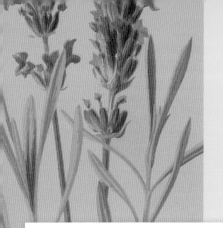

INTRODUCTION

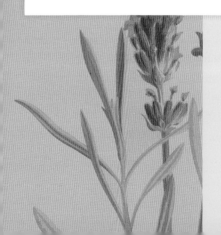

KALLIE'S STORY

The following true story, written by Kallie's mother, perfectly embodies the steps involved in emotional healing—from the time of trauma through the healing crisis and on to wholeness. It beautifully illustrates how the use of essential oils facilitates physical, emotional, and spiritual healing. We sincerely thank Kallie and her family for allowing their story to be told here.

When my daughter Kallie was two years old, she accidentally pulled a slow cooker full of boiling meat down onto herself, severely burning her face and torso. Second- and third-degree burns covered a third of her body. For a month, Kallie recuperated in a special burn unit where she received heavy narcotics along with other medications to help numb the intense pain that accompanies such severe burns. Two surgeries were necessary to place skin grafts on her face, neck, and shoulders. When Kallie finally came home, she had to wear a plastic mask on her face and a tight-fitting body suit for six months to keep the skin grafts from warping.

As her mother, it was horrifying to see my child suffer so much pain; I felt helpless. But Kallie was a very strong girl who tried her best to adapt to the excruciating medical procedures, such as having the dead skin scrubbed from the burned area or working through physical therapy. During the many times when the pain and trauma were too much for little Kallie, she would mentally leave us. I could see it in her hollow eyes. The first time I saw this was when the initial burn happened. In those few seconds right after the hot liquid touched her precious skin, she wasn't there. Due to the combination of heavy narcotics and unbearable procedures, she was physically and emotionally numb or just plain absent during most of the month that she was hospitalized. After we got home, it took a while to get back to regular life. Kallie was just so fragile and delicate. I tried my absolute best to physically and emotionally help her and our family recover from this event, but it was quite a challenge.

The months and years went by, and I started to notice that Kallie was extremely numb to pain. She was a very active, adventurous girl and had quite a few falls and injuries just like any other child, but she rarely acknowledged that it hurt her. Sometimes it was disturbing. I remember one visit to the doctor for her regular vaccines. Kallie lay down on the table, and the two nurses poked both her legs two times each. I watched her face and there was absolutely no physical or emotional reaction whatsoever. She was unfeeling. She often got nasty gashes or scrapes, and I wouldn't even know about them until later when I gave her a bath or changed her clothes. I would ask her where she got hurt and a lot of times she didn't even remember. She was also very self-conscious of the physical changes the burn had caused. When Kallie began school, she tried to hide her scars by covering them with her hair or coat or by walking with her face pointed toward the wall and away from onlookers.

I never pushed her to talk about it or do anything that was uncomfortable for her, but I gently tried to give her opportunities to share her thoughts and feelings. When Kallie was about five and a half, she started to forget what happened. She knew that something big occurred a long time ago, but she couldn't remember the details. Sometimes there was a trigger that sparked her memory, like the word "burn," or a fire, or even a bath. Then with fear and confusion in her eyes she would start asking, "What happened to me, Mom?" Around this time, I was introduced to essential oils. As my mother and I learned about the oils and their benefits, we thought of Kallie. Helichrysum and Vetiver seemed like the perfect fit, and we began treatment. I was so excited in the beginning, mostly thinking of the potential physical healing and largely unaware of the emotional benefits. Kallie was full of faith. She immediately said, "I know it's going to make my burn melt away, Mom!" I had no idea what was coming.

After only a few days of using the oils, Kallie started to act differently. The first thing I noticed was that she started to complain of physical pain for which we could find no reasonable explanation. Every time she would get the smallest cut or bruise, she had major anxiety about it—very opposite from her recent tough, numb-to-pain reactions. She cried for hours about tiny cuts or slivers and would say through tears, "Is it ever going to go away?" Kallie spent a large portion of the day worrying about the smallest things. It was almost impossible to convince her to take a bath. She became extremely picky about the clothes she wore. If clothing touched her "wrong" or was at all tight, she wouldn't wear it. Any mention of her being burned or even the word "burn" caused extreme fear. Anxiety attacks surfaced. Sometimes she randomly sat on my lap and just cried. I would cry too.

I finally realized Kallie was going through a healing crisis brought on by the oils. It made perfect sense. Every odd thing that she was doing directly correlated to the burn or to her experience in the hospital. With the help of essential oils, her body was expelling or ejecting all of the pain and hidden emotions that were buried for so long.

We guessed that the healing would probably last for the same amount of time she had stayed in the hospital. This was exactly right. It lasted a month. I tried my best to validate what she was feeling and to help her as much as I could during this time. I learned that if I missed a day of putting on her oils, it was a bad day for her and the rest of the household! So, I kept up with it and the results were phenomenal.

After this difficult month, I began to notice that words which had previously triggered a negative reaction from Kallie did not seem to bother her. She had a totally new and positive perspective. I could see plain as day that she was no longer coming from a place of fear. Instead of being self-conscious or shy, she was secure, strong, and confident—a totally different Kallie.

As her mom, I can see without a doubt that these essential oils gave her such a beautiful new outlook on herself and her past traumatic experience. On the morning of Kallie's seventh birthday, I was telling her about the day she was born, and she said, "I don't remember that, Mom, but I do remember when I was burned." I carefully asked, "What do you feel when you remember it?" She replied in her bubbly, secure voice, "Let me spell it for you mom: OK!" Words cannot express how very grateful I am that my little Kallie could heal emotionally.

FIVE STAGES OF HEALING

As illustrated in Kallie's story, essential oils play a powerful role in emotional healing. They lead us by the hand as we courageously face our emotional issues. Like Kallie, we all hold unresolved feelings of pain and hurt that long to be brought to the surface for transformation and healing.

Essential oils support healing in five stages. They strengthen us during each stage and prepare us for the next level of healing. For example, as we regain our physical health, we are invited to enter the emotional realm. In this manual, we briefly explore stages one, three, four, and five; however, the main focus of this book is stage two: the emotional stage.

FIVE STAGES OF HEALING:

1. Essential oils assist in healing the physical body.

2. Essential oils assist in healing the heart.

3. Essential oils assist in releasing limiting beliefs.

4. Essential oils increase spiritual awareness and connection.

5. Essential oils inspire the fulfillment of our life's purpose.

1. HEAL THE PHYSICAL BODY

Essential oils are powerful physical healers. Some essential oils are considered to be 40–60 times more potent than herbs.[1] Essential oils assist the body in fighting unfriendly microorganisms; purifying organs, glands, and body systems; balancing body functions; and raising the body's energetic vibration.[2]

2. HEAL THE HEART

As the oils support our physical health, they provide us with the energy needed to enter into the heart. Essential oils raise the vibration of the physical body.[3] As the body lives in higher energetic vibrations, lower energies (such as suppressed emotions) become unbearable. The body wants to release these feelings. Stagnant

anger, sadness, grief, judgment, and low
self-worth cannot exist in the environment of balance and peace
which essential oils help to create.

Emotional healing occurs as old feelings surface and release.[4]
Sometimes this experience is confused with regression. People may
perceive they are going backward or that the essential oils are not
working. We are so used to symptomatic healing that we have been
conditioned to view healing as the immediate cessation of all physical
and emotional pain. In reality, the oils are working. They are working
to permanently address emotional issues by supporting individuals
through their healing. Two key principles of healing the heart follow:

Release & Receive
It is important to understand that healing is a process. The process
can be separated into two main principles: release and receive.

We must release trapped negative emotions before we can receive
positive feelings. The old must go to make space for the new. We
often want to skip this step, but it is a necessary one. We must
be willing to experience the cleansing if we truly desire healing.
Resisting the cleansing process makes healing more painful. We
must surrender to the experience so that we may continue on the
path of healing. The more we let go and trust, the more enjoyable
this healing process can be.

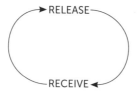

Essential Oils Don't Do Our Emotional Work for Us
Essential oils assist individuals in taking an honest look within. They
foster the right environment for healing, but they will not do the work
for us. In gardening, it is a common mistake to pull the weeds while
leaving the roots. This is particularly true for hard and rocky soils. To
ensure we uproot the whole plant, we can add water to the soil, which
allows the entire weed to be removed. Similarly, essential oils prepare

our emotional soil so that weeds may be removed with greater ease. However, they do not do the weeding for us. If we neglect to do the work of pulling our weeds, we have simply watered the problem. On the other hand, when we combine essential oils with emotional work, we reap the fruits of our labor.

3. RELEASE LIMITING BELIEFS

Unlike emotions, which are temporary in nature, beliefs are long term and deeply rooted in our subconscious. Beliefs are our deeply held framework that is forged from the conclusions we make about our experiences. This belief framework forms the lens through which we see life. For better or worse, our beliefs about ourselves are what we use to define our identity. This has far-reaching effects on all our behavior, thoughts, and emotional patterns. All of us have positive and negative beliefs. However, our negative or limiting beliefs can cause the same issues to reoccur over and over throughout our lives. Repeated experiences reinforce the associated emotional pathways. Essential oils assist in illuminating the emotional patterns of deeply held beliefs, encouraging us to identify what the limiting beliefs are, releasing the trapped energy and associated emotions, and, finally, replacing them with positive beliefs that will serve our highest good.

4. INCREASE SPIRITUAL AWARENESS & CONNECTION

All beings were created with divine intention. Acknowledgment of our spiritual nature and connection to our source is an essential part of healing. Most important in this stage is the awareness of that intention and the infinite love available to us. It is from this love that our healing can become more complete.

5. INSPIRE FULFILLMENT OF LIFE'S PURPOSE

When we have experienced the previous four aspects—essential to heal holistically—we are now ready to fully actualize our purpose and potential. This stage is where we achieve the clarity and courage to follow the path meant for us.

1. Schnaubelt, K. (2011). *The Healing Intelligence of Essential Oils.* (pp. 13-16). Rochester, VT: Healing Arts Press.

2. Stewart, D. (2003). *Healing Oils of the Bible.* (pp. 31-34). Marble Hill, MO: Care Publications.

3. Stewart, D. (pp. 31-34).

4. Moreton, V. S. (1992). *A New Day in Healing!* (pp. 16-17). San Diego, CA: Kalos Publishing.

DECODING EMOTIONS

Tuning In to the Mind-Body Connection

Identifying the exact emotions you are experiencing at any given moment can sometimes be challenging. You know that you're feeling something but may not know exactly what. Thankfully, emotions are experienced throughout the entire body, so we can look to it for clues.

Our brain's limbic system governs our emotional responses and sends different chemical messages for the different emotions we experience. Our body has specific physical reactions to the various chemical messages, thus providing an indication as to the emotion that triggered them. For example, "stressed" is an emotional state that generally causes the release of extra adrenaline and cortisol. Those chemicals trigger physical reactions such as increased heart rate, changes in breathing, trembling, digestive upset, perspiration, and so on. If you're experiencing a combination of these symptoms, there's a good chance the emotion you're experiencing is "stressed."

Though there are some general reactions that give us a fairly predictable foundation, it's possible to experience multiple feelings simultaneously. For example, when we feel threatened, we often feel anger and fear at the same time. Additionally, physical responses to very different emotions can feel quite similar. For example, the physical indicators of being terrified and exhilarated are largely the same. The brain, in context with our individual experiences and beliefs, will shape which emotion we feel and how.

While the experience of emotions can be as varied as the people having them, the following chart provides some examples of physical indicators commonly associated with the emotions listed.

Reference the following chart for a brief overview of emotions and corresponding physical indicators.

EMOTION	ASSOCIATED EMOTIONS	PHYSICAL INDICATOR	MENTAL OR EMOTIONAL INDICATOR
FEAR	Anxious Irritable Prideful Judgmental Scarcity Jealous Weak Vulnerable Controlling Unsafe	• Rapid or shallow breathing • Increased heart rate • Blood draining from face or limbs • Nausea • Throat contraction • Clenching or tightening in chest or stomach • Sweaty palms • Dizziness • Butterflies or fluttering in stomach • Muscle weakness	• Unsure • Uneasy • Restless • Hesitant • Panicked • Terrified • Phobias • Apprehensive • Paranoid • Worried • Unable to concentrate • Dreading • Preoccupied with future events or other people's behavior
HAPPINESS	Content Joyful Excited Optimistic	• Warmth starting from the inside and radiating out, sometimes centered around chest • Physical relaxation, or increased energy • Feeling of expansiveness • Breathing deeper, and easier mental clarity	• Pleasant thoughts and feelings • Content • Satisfied • Safe • Elated • Positive • Enthusiastic • Vibrant • Buoyant • Cheerful • Serene • Sense of well-being • Hopeful

EMOTION	ASSOCIATED EMOTIONS	PHYSICAL INDICATOR	MENTAL OR EMOTIONAL INDICATOR
ANGER	Frustrated Resentful Irritated Incensed Raging Hateful	• Tightness of muscles • Pain or pressure in back • Neck, and jaw • Feeling hot • Adrenaline response including increased sensation in arms and hands • Increased heart rate and blood pressure • Shaking or trembling • Sweating	• Escalation of powerful, intense, or suppressed feelings • Masking fear or sadness • Explosive outburst • Withdrawn • Silent • Defensive or blaming • Resentful • Irritated, sarcastic, or cynical
LOVE	Passionate Fond Forgiving Compassionate Empathetic Caring	Love can be a total physical experience, generally with • Increased blood flow and • Warmth often felt primarily in chest	• Content • Strong affection • Feeling complete or filled • Compassionate • General well-being • Bonded • Observant • Selfless desires and actions
SADNESS	Hurting Sorrowful Loss Grieving Lonely	• Heaviness in chest • Lump in throat • Crying • Aches and pains • Lethargy • Fatigue	• Heavy • Down • Blue • Apathetic • Betrayed • Isolated • Sorrowful • Anguished • Hopeless or despairing

EMOTION	ASSOCIATED EMOTIONS	PHYSICAL INDICATOR	MENTAL OR EMOTIONAL INDICATOR
PEACE	Present Grounded Content	• Relaxation in muscle tension especially in face and upper torso • Cessation or reduction of pain • Warmth through body • Reduced pulse • Steady breathing	• Calm • Relaxed • Patient • Content • Connection • Serene • Flexible • Accepting • Untroubled • Purposeful
GUILT	Shameful Regretful Self-loathing	• Tightening or aching sensations in stomach and chest • Other uncomfortable sensations in head and face as well as lower abdomen	• Fearful • Angry • Sad • Regretful • Desire to run away or disappear • Avoiding or denying • Embarrassed • Feeling like a failure or worthless
STRESS	Overwhelmed Unsupported Controlled Overworked Burned out Obligated	• Muscle tension in shoulders neck, and head • Overly alert or difficulty concentrating • Headaches • Indigestion or nausea • Rapid breathing • General aches and pains • Heart palpitations • Changes in eating and sleep habits	• Feeling pressured by people or circumstances • Depleted • Drained • Overwhelmed • Burdened • Anxious • Fearful • Angry • Sad • Hopeless • Noticeable changes in mood or behavior such as being withdrawn, indecisive, and tearful; or suddenly reactive, irritable, and lashing out

TOOLS FOR EMOTIONAL WORK

There are several great aids to assist you when beginning your emotional work. We suggest that you integrate these tools with essential oils to facilitate the healing process.

MEDITATION

Regardless of method, most mindfulness-based practices have a positive effect on mental and emotional well-being. Choose any method that resonates with you and practice it consistently to enhance the benefits of all other emotional healing practices. Meditation practitioners find that the benefits are compounded over time.

JOURNALING

Keeping any kind of journal can be beneficial. Three main journaling techniques include keeping a gratitude journal; free writing (or stream-of-consciousness journaling); or letter writing, where you work out your feelings in a letter to someone (not necessarily to be mailed). Writing your thoughts and feelings eases mental strain, releases stagnant energy, lifts dark moods, inspires creative and diverse thought, increases self-worth, and invites calm. It's a powerful tool for processing all types of emotional experiences.

PERSONAL INVENTORY

This time-honored technique involves making a self-assessment: listing personal strengths and positive qualities on one side of a chart and weaknesses or blocks to success on the other. This will help you acknowledge what's working in your life (often the most important part of the process) and help you to identify what's out of balance. A deep and honest moral inventory is part of most twelve-step recovery programs.

NATURE THERAPY

Recent science is reporting that significant benefits come from spending time outdoors in any context from exercising to relaxing to meditating. Walking barefoot in grass or sand, putting your hands in soil, strolling in natural areas with lots of trees—even watching beautiful nature films or art portraying nature—can make you feel grounded, centered, and more at peace.

PERSONALIZED MODALITIES

From music therapy, play therapy, and talk therapy to energy work, regression work, and subconscious work, there are a variety of modalities and therapies that can assist emotional healing and recovery. Feel free to pair essential oils with any practice that serves you.

HEALTH HABITS

Additionally, all emotional work is enhanced by building on a strong base of physical health. You don't need to wait until you have faultless physical health habits in order to begin. Try to give yourself the nutrition, exercise, and especially the sleep that you need, and you will see even greater benefits from your essential oils.

HOW TO USE ESSENTIAL OILS

Please reference all safety information from the manufacturer or a reliable reference book when using essential oils for aromatic, topical, or internal use.

AROMATIC

To use an essential oil aromatically, simply smell the oil directly from the bottle. Or place a few drops into a diffuser, which disperses the oil into the air. Another option is to add a few drops into the palms of the hands, rub together, and inhale.

TOPICAL

To use an essential oil topically, add a few drops in the palm of the hand with a carrier oil and apply to desired area. Essential oils are very potent, so a small amount should be sufficient. Due to their volatility (rapid evaporation), diluting essential oils with a carrier oil is recommended; dilution is especially recommended for those with sensitive skin, including children and babies. Dilution does not reduce efficacy; rather it may increase absorption. If you are pregnant or nursing, pay close attention to your body and decrease use with sensitivities. Consult a physician as necessary.

INTERNAL

Only use Certified Pure Therapeutic Grade® essential oils if you take an essential oil internally. Place a few drops under your tongue, in a gel capsule, or in a glass of water. Children may prefer the essential oil added to honey for their internal use.

Certified Pure Therapeutic Grade® oils are tested at independent laboratories with gas chromatography, mass spectrometry, and numerous other tests to verify their purity and composition. CPTG® oils that meet these rigorous testing standards are safe for aromatic, topical, and internal use by all ages. Only the highest-quality and purest essential oils should be used for physical, emotional, and spiritual healing. In this guide, we have chosen to focus in on dōTERRA's CPTG® essential oils.

HOW TO USE THIS BOOK

OIL DESCRIPTIONS

Essential oils are highly concentrated versions of the powerful natural oils found in various parts of plants. These symbols indicate the specific origin of the single oils included in this book.

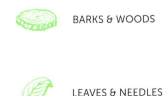 BARKS & WOODS

 PEELS

 LEAVES & NEEDLES

 FLOWERS

 RESINS

 ROOTS

 SEEDS

FRUITS & BERRIES

The main body of this manual is divided into individual descriptions of the oils. Single oils are listed first followed by blends. Read the descriptions to determine which essential oil is best suited for your emotional needs.

BODY GUIDE

If you're unsure how to identify which emotion you are feeling, start in Decoding Emotions to match up your physical and emotional symptoms.

EMOTIONS GUIDE

You can search the comprehensive Emotions Guide to find specific emotional states and recommended oils to support those states. Use the Negative Emotions and Positive Properties chart for a quick overview of the emotions and properties related to each oil.

ESSENTIAL EMOTIONS WHEEL

For quick reference, refer to the wheel (available separately). One side lists negative emotions (what you would like less of in your life) and the other side lists positive properties (what you would like more of in your life). When you find the emotion or property that resonates with you, read the oil description in this book for a more complete understanding.

ESSENTIAL EMOTIONS APP

While you're on the go, look up emotions, body part, or oil. Available for both iOS and Android.

The app and the book are coming in the following languages: Spanish, Chinese, Dutch, French , German, Hungarian, Italian, Korean, Portuguese, Romanian, and Russian.

ESSENTIAL OIL REFERENCE GUIDES

This guide may also be used as a companion to essential oil reference guides focused on physical health and use. After finding the recommended oils for your physical condition, cross-reference the oils with the emotional descriptions here. For the most powerful results, choose the oils that match your emotional state as well as your physical condition.

SCANNING TECHNOLOGIES

This book serves as an excellent companion with scanning technologies that recommend a customized oil regimen for physical as well as emotional healing.

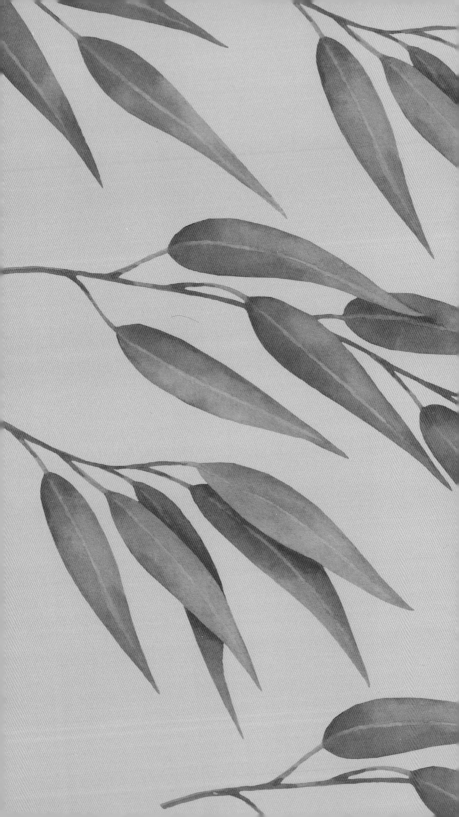

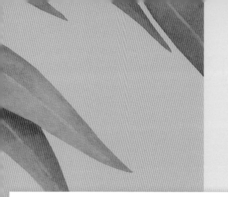

SINGLE OILS

This section is the core emotional properties of each essential oil. These descriptions briefly summarize the fruits of our research. The process for determining the focus of each oil includes gathering research on essential oils (e.g., their botanical and medicinal properties, plant family characteristics, history, and cultivation). The characteristics of each oil are also manifested through personal and professional experience. In the final analysis, the representation of each oil has also been guided and influenced by intuitive and energetic learning.

In each description is the oil's emotional purpose summarized in the subtitle, which honors the emotional characteristics most prevalent in the oil. Both positive properties encouraged by the oil and the negative emotions addressed by the oil are listed, as well as companion oils. The companion oils are provided to complement the primary properties of the oil. While the emotional stories of each person are varied, these complementary oils support the core emotional state and provide alternatives for additional research and reflection.

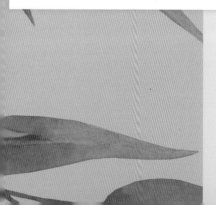

ARBORVITAE
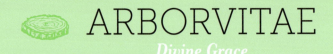
Divine Grace

Arborvitae assists individuals who believe or act like all progress must be made through struggle and solitary effort. Instead of trusting in the Divine, these individuals unconsciously block divine aid, choosing instead to live by their own efforts. Arborvitae addresses the need to control one's outcomes in life. It invites individuals to live with peace and joy by trusting in the abundant flow of divine grace.

Arborvitae is also a grounding oil that teaches Divinity is all around. God's grace can be felt and experienced here on earth; it is not distant or separate. God can help find balance in life and teach what to hold close and what to release.

Arborvitae's Latin name means "to sacrifice." This oil invites individuals to sacrifice their personal will and ambitions for a far more fulfilling way of living. By surrendering to God, the mind relaxes and the soul experiences harmony and peace. Arborvitae teaches that true strength can come through emptiness or a willingness to receive God's strength. It asks individuals to relax, take a deep breath, and trust in the flow of life. Arborvitae assists the soul to live effortlessly by divine grace.

NEGATIVE EMOTIONS: Willful, excessive effort, distrusting, rigid, fearful, controlling

POSITIVE PROPERTIES: Peaceful, surrender, grounded, trusting, relaxed, grace

COMPANION OILS: Basil, Cilantro, Oregano, Copaiba, Cumin, Hinoki

SUGGESTED USES:
Aromatic: Inhale from bottle, diffuse, or place drops in hand, rub, and inhale.

Topical: Apply 1-3 drops over solar plexus (upper stomach), on crown of head, or bottom of feet.

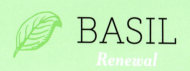

BASIL

Renewal

The symptoms of adrenal exhaustion help identify the main moods that are improved with Basil, primarily fatigue, low energy, being overwhelmed, and the inability to cope with life's stressors. The smell of Basil oil brings strength to the heart and relaxation to the mind. This oil is also excellent for states of nervousness, anxiousness, and despair.

Basil oil supports those who are under a great deal of mental strain. It brings rejuvenation of vital forces after long periods of burnout and exhaustion. Basil oil may strengthen the adrenals and restore the body to its natural rhythms of sleep, activity, and rest.

Basil oil is also helpful for recovery from negative habits. It gives hope and optimism to the tired soul. Basil may assist an individual in giving up false stimulants. By increasing natural energy, it helps individuals to achieve greater balance and health. In short, Basil is indicated for those who are weary in mind and body and for those in need of strength and renewal.

NEGATIVE EMOTIONS: Anxious, overwhelmed, drained, exhausted, negative habits

POSITIVE PROPERTIES: Energized, renewed, rejuvenated, rested, strengthened

COMPANION OILS: Wild Orange, Peppermint, Serenity®, Grapefruit, Cumin, DigestZen®, Red Mandarin, PastTense®, Tulsi

SUGGESTED USES:

Aromatic: Inhale from bottle, diffuse, or place drops in hand, rub, and inhale.

Topical: Apply 3-5 drops over adrenal glands (lower back) or on bottom of feet in the morning and before bed.

Internal: Take 1-2 drops under the tongue, in a capsule, or in water.

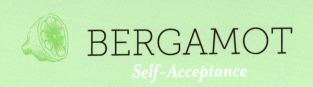

BERGAMOT
Self-Acceptance

Bergamot relieves feelings of despair, self-judgment, and low self-esteem. It supports individuals in need of self-acceptance and self-love. Bergamot invites individuals to see life with more optimism.

Bergamot has a cleansing effect on stagnant feelings and limiting belief systems. Because of core beliefs of being bad, unlovable, and not good enough, they seek to hide behind a facade of cheerfulness. They may fear revealing their true thoughts and feelings. Bergamot's powerful cleansing properties generate movement in the energy system, which in turn brings hope.

In this way, Bergamot is wonderful for those who feel down and hopeless. It awakens the soul to hope and offers courage to share the inner self. Reigniting optimism and confidence in the self, it imparts true self-acceptance. Bergamot teaches individuals to let go of self-judgment by learning to love themselves unconditionally.

NEGATIVE EMOTIONS: Despairing, low self-esteem, self-judgment, unlovable, hopeless

POSITIVE PROPERTIES: Self-acceptance, optimistic, confident, hopeful, lovable, good enough

COMPANION OILS: Cassia, Slim & Sassy®, Kumquat, Grapefruit, Copaiba, Beautiful, Pink Pepper, Bergamot Mint

SUGGESTED USES:

Aromatic: Inhale from bottle or diffuse.

Topical: Dilute 1-3 drops with carrier oil and apply over heart, solar plexus (upper stomach), or on forehead.

Internal: Take 1-2 drops under the tongue, in a capsule, or in water.

BERGAMOT MINT
Revived Heart

Bergamot Mint is primarily a heart-revitalizing oil. It is both beautifully uplifting and tenderly calming to the senses. It has a balancing effect on the emotions, comforting and soothing individuals when they feel like their heart is weighed down by the disappointments of life. It lifts them and helps them know they will heal and rise again.

Bergamot Mint opens up the soul to gentle inspiration followed by calm. It is a lovely oil for peaceful meditation or tranquil contemplation. This oil aids in simplifying problems that have grown out of proportion and are consuming too much emotional energy. It is also helpful when an individual's mind and heart are in need of deep, restorative rest.

Bergamot Mint encourages individuals to consciously consider if they are welcome in their own heart. It invites them to come home to themselves and be inspired from within. Its aroma reopens obscured and forgotten passageways, creating a welcoming refuge deep within their being. This oil facilitates complete self-acceptance so that the heart may unfold radiant, open, and alive.

NEGATIVE EMOTIONS: Weighed down, disappointed, rejection of self, closed to love, exhausted

POSITIVE PROPERTIES: Uplifted, hopeful, self-acceptance, loving, refreshed, open

COMPANION OILS: Rose, Lavender, Ylang Ylang, Helichrysum, Bergamot, Peppermint, Geranium, Lime, Cedarwood

SUGGESTED USES:

Aromatic: Inhale from bottle, diffuse, or place drops in hand, rub, and inhale.

Topical: Dilute 1 drop with carrier oil and apply over heart and on arms.

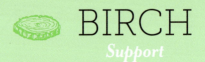

BIRCH

Support

Birch offers support to the unsupported. When a person is feeling attacked or unsupported in life, this oil offers courage to move forward alone. It helps individuals ground within their own center to find their source of inner support and strength. Learning to be flexible is important but so is gaining a strong backbone. Birch offers support to the weak-willed to stand tall and firm in what they believe, especially in situations where one is at risk of being rejected if they choose a different way. Birch lends its spirit of endurance to help individuals face trials of adversity, so they may weather storms with the strength and conviction of a tree.

Birch also encourages individuals to accept support when it is offered. Often, when individuals have carried their burdens alone, they don't know how to receive assistance. Birch counsels individuals to not become the reason they are unsupported, by blocking those who would lend their support. It reminds that it sometimes requires more strength to accept help than to go it alone.

Birch teaches those in need to trust that even if they are abandoned by all others, the Divine will always be there. It also reinforces there is more to life than pain, and with the right support and the right grounding, one can be held up and sustained through hardship.

NEGATIVE EMOTIONS: Unsupported, alienated, fearful, weak-willed, overly flexible, rejecting help

POSITIVE PROPERTIES: Supported, firm, resolute, strengthened, grounded, connected, receiving

COMPANION OILS: Cedarwood, White Fir, Coriander

SUGGESTED USES:
Aromatic: Inhale from bottle or diffuse.

Topical: Dilute 1-3 drops with carrier oil and apply along spine, over lower back, or on bottom of feet.

Internal: Take 1-2 drops under the tongue, in a capsule, or in water.

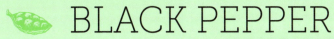

BLACK PEPPER
Unmasking

Black Pepper reveals the masks and facades used to hide aspects of the self. Since childhood, most individuals have been taught that some feelings and behaviors are good while others are not. So instead of seeking to understand seemingly inappropriate feelings and behaviors, they usually judge, condemn, and repress them. Individuals learn early on that to be loved and accepted, they must hide undesirable aspects of themselves behind a mask or facade.

Black Pepper invites individuals to get real by digging deep within the less understood parts of the self. Whether one's true motives and feelings are acknowledged or not, they continue to exist. The more these feelings are pushed down, buried, and repressed, the more they seek to make themselves known. If they are not honestly dealt with and acknowledged, they will often be expressed through erratic, compulsive, or addictive behaviors.

Black Pepper also reignites the soul fire, fueling motivation and high energy, and hastening the healing process. It gives individuals strength to overcome the challenges and issues they carry inside and invites them to live in integrity with their True Self.

NEGATIVE EMOTIONS: Emotionally dishonest, repressed emotions, trapped, prideful, superficial

POSITIVE PROPERTIES: Emotionally honest, authentic, courageous, motivated, self-aware, integrity

COMPANION OILS: Kumquat, Vetiver, Coriander, Juniper Berry, Frankincense, Pink Pepper

SUGGESTED USES:
Aromatic: Inhale from bottle or diffuse.

Topical: Dilute 1-2 drops with carrier oil and apply on bottom of feet.

Internal: Take 1-2 drops under the tongue, in a capsule, or in water.

BLACK SPRUCE
Stability

Black Spruce is both grounding and stabilizing. Of all the grounding oils, the spruces are the most effective. Spruces are especially helpful in times of crisis, shock, or trauma. During such experiences, a person's energy may splinter, causing emotional disruption. These trees stabilize an individual's energy, helping them return to a grounded, balanced state.

Black Spruce has mastered the art of energy conservation and endurance. It teaches individuals how to regulate their physical energy by listening to their body's rhythms and needs. Black Spruce models how to persevere through the storms of life by drawing strength from one's roots. It offers a model of vitality and longevity through living in harmony with nature's cycles and seasons. Spruce can also assist individuals who feel depleted of energy to renew themselves. It helps those who struggle with extreme moods to find balance and moderation.

Black Spruce is an ally in dealing with fear, especially sub-conscious, generational fears. All individuals hold genetic and DNA memories from the generations who have gone on before. At times, individuals may struggle under the weight of fears that didn't originate with them. Black Spruce helps them gain clarity about fear-based memories and release them from the mind and body—freeing themselves and others in the process.

NEGATIVE EMOTIONS: Unstable, depleted, fearful, exhausted, dysfunctional generational patterns

POSITIVE PROPERTIES: Stable, resolute, grounded, enduring, balanced

COMPANION OILS: Balance®, Holiday Peace®, Juniper Berry, Douglas Fir, Cedarwood, Vetiver, Island Mint®

SUGGESTED USES:
Aromatic: Inhale from bottle, diffuse, or place drops in hand, rub, and inhale.

Topical: Apply to lower back, across forehead, or on bottom of feet.

BLUE TANSY

Inspired Action

Blue Tansy supports those who resist taking action to change or transform their circumstances. It is especially helpful when individuals have become stagnant in their progression. It provides a kind of catalytic spark that overcomes the tendency to vacillate, avoid, or procrastinate. Blue Tansy necessitates that individuals choose to take the helm of their life. It also encourages individuals to live in alignment with the whisperings of their inner voice, prompting them to make necessary changes. When an individual represses these messages, they often feel lethargic, drained, apathetic, sluggish, and exhausted. Blue Tansy invites individuals to take the initiative to reclaim the life they dream of.

Blue Tansy invites individuals to manifest their passion into action. This is especially important when there is a desire to retreat or self-sabotage. By creating more inward mobility, Blue Tansy encourages them to accept all that is, including emotional setbacks and other challenges which must be overcome to actualize inspiration and sustain change. Blue Tansy teaches that each act is based on choice and requires individuals to own the responsibility of their cumulative choices. It demands personal mastery and purposeful action in achieving one's fullest potential.

NEGATIVE EMOTIONS: Procrastinating, resisting change and inner guidance, uninspired, exhausted, lethargic, apathetic, self-sabotage

POSITIVE PROPERTIES: Inspired, initiative, committed, responsive, energized, motivated, purposeful, responsible

COMPANION OILS: Litsea, Coriander, Roman Chamomile, Fennel, Turmeric, Laurel Leaf

SUGGESTED USES:
Aromatic: Inhale from bottle or diffuse.

Topical: Dilute 1-3 drops with carrier oil and apply behind ears, on wrists, over solar plexus (upper stomach), or on bottom of feet.

CARDAMOM
Objectivity

Cardamom helps individuals to regain objectivity, mental sobriety, and self-control. It assists individuals who frequently feel frustrated or angry with other people. Cardamom is especially helpful for times when one's anger goes to their head, causing them to become hotheaded. In such situations, the individual becomes inebriated with anger, losing control and rational function. Cardamom helps to bring balance, mental clarity, and objectivity during moments of extreme anger and frustration.

Cardamom is especially beneficial for individuals with a long history of anger or aggression, which often becomes directed outward. It is helpful for those who hyperfocus on their problems, especially their frustrations. Cardamom assists individuals in breaking down or digesting these intense emotions of frustration and anger by redirecting energy to the solar plexus, the center of responsibility. In this way, Cardamom helps individuals let go of emotional distortions which cause them to objectify other people and see them as inconveniences.

Cardamom demands that individuals stop blaming others. It asks them to take personal ownership and responsibility for their feelings. As they do, they will feel more at peace, calm, and in control of themselves.

NEGATIVE EMOTIONS: Inebriated by anger, easily frustrated, objectifying others, blaming, unable to think clearly

POSITIVE PROPERTIES: Objective, self-control, respectful, tolerant, patient, mental sobriety

COMPANION OILS: Thyme, Serenity®, Oregano, Niaouli

SUGGESTED USES:
Aromatic: Inhale from bottle or diffuse.

Topical: Dilute 1-2 drops with carrier oil and apply anywhere anger is held in the body.

Internal: Take 1-2 drops under the tongue, in a capsule, or in water.

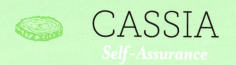

CASSIA
Self-Assurance

Cassia brings gladness and courage to the heart and soul. It is a wonderful remedy for the shy and timid. It helps those who hold back and try to hide. When a person avoids being the center of attention, Cassia can restore their confidence.

Similar to Cinnamon, Cassia dispels fear and replaces it with self-assurance. It challenges individuals to try, even when they are afraid of making mistakes. Cassia aids those who feel foolish by helping them see their own brilliance. It supports the soul in seeing its own value and potential. Cassia assists individuals in discovering their innate gifts and talents. It invites them to let their light shine and live from their True Self.

NEGATIVE EMOTIONS: Embarrassed, hiding, fearful, humiliated, insecure, judged, shy, worthless

POSITIVE PROPERTIES: Courageous, self-assured, unashamed, confident, valued, authentic

COMPANION OILS: Spearmint, Clove, Roman Chamomile, Litsea, Beautiful, Pink Pepper, Star Anise, Turmeric, Laurel Leaf

SUGGESTED USES:
Aromatic: Inhale from bottle or diffuse.

Topical: Dilute 1 drop or less with carrier oil and apply over solar plexus (upper stomach) or on bottom of feet. **NOTE:** Use caution when applying topically.

Internal: Take 1-2 drops under the tongue, in a capsule, or in water.

CEDARWOOD
Community

Cedarwood brings people together to experience the strength and value of community. Those in need of Cedarwood struggle to form bonds within social groups. This can often be due to an overdeveloped sense of individuality. Rather than allowing themselves to be supported by family, friends, or a community, they live by excessive self-reliance. On the other hand, the individual's difficulty forming social roots may also stem from feeling disconnected and separate from the human family. Cedarwood inspires the feeling of belonging and assists the heart in opening to receive the love and support of other people. It invites the strong-willed individual to couple the strength of individuality with the supportive power of community.

Cedarwood supports individuals in seeing that they are not alone; life is a shared experience. Cedarwood also assists in opening the awareness of individuals to the support system that is already available to them, such as friends or family that have been overlooked. It invites individuals to both give and receive, so they may experience the strength of groups and the joy of relationships.

NEGATIVE EMOTIONS: Inability to form social bonds, lonely, feeling separate from the human family, antisocial

POSITIVE PROPERTIES: Emotionally connected, belonging, supported, social bonds, sociable, community oriented

COMPANION OILS: Marjoram, Birch, Magnolia

SUGGESTED USES:
Aromatic: Inhale from bottle or diffuse.

Topical: Dilute 3-4 drops with carrier oil and apply on arms, legs, or bottom of feet.

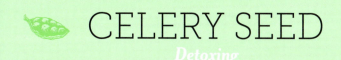

CELERY SEED
Detoxing

Celery is a traditional detoxifying and cleansing remedy needed for a modern age. Never before has the entire earth been more drenched in toxic substances, in the air, water, and soil. Even daily media consumption is filled with toxicity toward hearts and minds. Human bodies are struggling to cope with the onslaught to their detoxification pathways. This pestilent barrage wears down the body's natural ability to purge both emotional and physical toxins. Celery will partner with individuals when they know they must journey into an emotional or physical detox to restore their internal equilibrium.

Celery invites individuals to straighten their course and return to practices that will lead to better outcomes. It teaches that cleansing the inner vessel requires ongoing commitment, and perseverance, oftentimes rejecting what comes easily in favor of what is necessary. It promotes greater alignment within an individual's heart and body, and the discovery of personal solutions that are sustainable. Celery aids individuals in releasing anything that is not supporting their wellness and well-being.

NEGATIVE EMOTIONS: Toxic, sluggish, stagnant, imbalanced, unhealthy

POSITIVE PROPERTIES: Restored, cleansed, well, balanced, realigned, committed

COMPANION OILS: Cilantro, Lemongrass, Lemon Myrtle, Lime, Purify, Zendocrine®, DDR Prime®

SUGGESTED USES:
Aromatic: Inhale from bottle, diffuse, or place drops in hand, rub, and inhale.

Topical: Apply on bottom of feet.

Internal: Take 1-2 drops under the tongue, in a capsule, or in water.

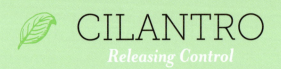

CILANTRO
Releasing Control

Cilantro facilitates a detoxification of negative emotions and debris. It is helpful in lightening one's load through the release of issues buried in the body, heart, and soul. Similar to Coriander oil, which is distilled from the seeds of the same plant, Cilantro assists individuals in shedding what is not in harmony with their True Self.

Those in need of Cilantro may attempt to obsessively control other people or manage their environment. Inwardly, these individuals may experience a great deal of worry and mental strain. They may become constricted, clinging to or obsessing over material possessions. Individuals may even hold onto the very patterns, emotions, issues, and possessions that may impair or betray their True Self.

Cilantro facilitates emotional cleansing, and especially encourages the release of worry and control as it assists individuals in centering in their True Self. Cilantro liberates the soul from heavy burdens, enabling the individual to live light and free.

NEGATIVE EMOTIONS: Controlling, toxic, constricted, obsessive-compulsive, clingy, worried, trapped

POSITIVE PROPERTIES: Cleansing, liberated, detached, untroubled

COMPANION OILS: Wintergreen, Cypress, Cinnamon, Peace®, Cardamom

SUGGESTED USES:
Aromatic: Inhale from bottle, diffuse, or place drops in hand, rub, and inhale.

Topical: Apply 1-3 drops over throat or solar plexus (upper stomach).

Internal: Take 1-2 drops under the tongue, in a capsule, or in water.

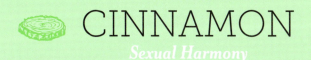

CINNAMON
Sexual Harmony

Cinnamon supports sexual issues and the reproductive system. It assists individuals in accepting their body and embracing their physical attractiveness. Cinnamon dispels fear of rejection and nurtures healthy sexuality. It rekindles sexual energies when there has been repression, trauma, or abuse. It can also bring clarity to souls who struggle with their sexual identity.

Cinnamon also assists individuals in relationships where insecurities are shown by jealousy or control. It encourages the soul to let go of control and allow others to be free. Cinnamon can nurture strong relationships based on mutual love and respect. Where there are other insecurities covered by pretense, facade, and pride, Cinnamon warms and bolsters individuals helping them feel safe, protected, and secure enough to choose humility and risk being truly known. Cinnamon invites individuals to be honest and vulnerable, thereby allowing true intimacy to emerge.

NEGATIVE EMOTIONS: Body shame, fearful, controlling, jealous, sexual issues, sexual repression or overactive sexuality

POSITIVE PROPERTIES: Body acceptance, attractive, accepted, healthy sexuality, intimate

COMPANION OILS: Jasmine, Bergamot, Grapefruit, Neroli

SUGGESTED USES:
Aromatic: Inhale from bottle or diffuse.

Topical: Dilute 1 drop or less with carrier oil and apply over sacral chakra (lower stomach). **NOTE:** Use caution when applying topically.

Internal: Take 1-2 drops under the tongue, in a capsule, or in water.

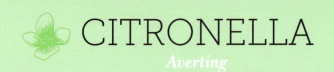

CITRONELLA
Averting

Citronella is potent for repelling unwanted invaders from the body and energy field. While it's best to try and avert invasion or contamination from harmful organisms or energies, it is not always possible. Citronella also assists individuals in expelling undesirables once they have been established.

The invitation from Citronella is to carefully observe what individuals are allowing into their physical, mental, and emotional space and to choose more consciously what they allow into their lives. It reminds that small weeds grow quickly when left unattended.

Citronella is especially helpful when individuals have been unconsciously allowing little irritations and judgments to build up over time. Recurring negative thoughts and reactions accumulate and stagnate in various parts of the body, causing havoc. Citronella challenges individuals to reckon with their addiction to feeling agitated and annoyed. It assists in breaking the energetic cycle of constant irritation and teaches how to release these degrading states so they don't continue to prey on the life force.

NEGATIVE EMOTIONS: Irritated, judgmental, invaded, overrun, undiscerning, stagnant

POSITIVE PROPERTIES: Averting, discerning, forgiving, releasing, repelling

COMPANION OILS: Lemongrass, Lemon Eucalyptus, Forgive®, Thyme, Cardamom, Niaouli

SUGGESTED USES:
Aromatic: Inhale from bottle, diffuse, or place drops in hand, rub, and inhale.

Topical: Dilute 1-2 drops with carrier oil and apply on bottom of feet.

Environmental: Add several drops into spray bottle and mist around home.

CLARY SAGE
Clarity & Vision

Clary Sage assists individuals in changing their perceptions. It gives courage to see the truth. One of the finest oils for the brow chakra, Clary Sage dispels darkness and illusion, helping individuals to see their limiting belief systems. Clary Sage encourages individuals to remain open to new ideas and new perspectives. It can assist during a healing crisis when a drastic change of perspective is required. Clary Sage opens the soul to new possibilities and experiences.

Clary Sage assists in opening creative channels and clearing creative blocks. It eliminates distractions from the mind and assists individuals in finding a state of emptiness where creative forces may be realized. Opening individuals to the dream world, Clary Sage increases the ability to visualize and imagine new possibilities.

Clary Sage teaches the spirit how to use its divinely given gifts and is especially helpful in clarifying spiritual vision. It assists in developing the gift of discernment. Clary Sage invites individuals to expand their vision and accept the reality of the spiritual world.

NEGATIVE EMOTIONS: Confused, darkness, spiritually disconnected, hopeless, blocked creativity

POSITIVE PROPERTIES: Spiritual clarity, intuitive, open-minded, imaginative, spiritually discerning

COMPANION OILS: Lemongrass, Black Pepper, Juniper Berry, Rosemary, Melissa, Davana, Tulsi

SUGGESTED USES:
Aromatic: Inhale from bottle, diffuse, or place drops in hand, rub, and inhale.

Topical: Apply 1-2 drops on forehead or behind ears.

Internal: Take 1-2 drops under the tongue, in a capsule, or in water.

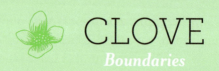

CLOVE
Boundaries

Clove supports individuals in letting go of victim mentality. Victims feel overly influenced by other people and outside circumstances. They perceive themselves as powerless to change their life situations. Clove helps individuals stand up for themselves, be proactive, and feel capable of making their own choices, regardless of others.

Clove assists individuals in letting go of patterns of self-betrayal and codependency by reconnecting them with their personal integrity. It builds up appropriate boundaries and defenses. Clove gives pushovers the courage to say no. It reignites the inner fire and encourages individuals to stand up for themselves. It can assist when there has been a history of weakened boundaries caused by mistreatment, exploitation, repeated traumatic or compromising experiences. Clove is helpful in breaking free of these patterns by restoring the sense of self and helping individuals regain the strength needed to advocate for their right to self-containment and protection.

NEGATIVE EMOTIONS: Victim mentality, defeated, dominated, enslaved, fear of rejection, intimidated, controlled, codependent

POSITIVE PROPERTIES: Empowered, clear boundaries, protected, courageous, independent, capable, proactive, integrity

COMPANION OILS: Ginger, Helichrysum, Tea Tree, Coriander

SUGGESTED USES:
Aromatic: Inhale from bottle or diffuse.

Topical: Dilute 1 drop or less with carrier oil and apply on bottom of feet or over sacral chakra (lower stomach). **NOTE:** Use caution when applying topically.

Internal: Take 1-2 drops under the tongue, in a capsule, or in water.

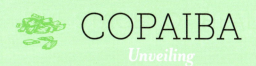

COPAIBA
Unveiling

Copaiba invites individuals to connect with their past. It offers a deep intertwining energy that links experience to experience to unveil the deeper meaning and messages showing up in one's life. Copaiba respects the sacred sheltered within until it is ready to emerge into the light of consciousness. It then invites individuals to become thoughtfully aware of the shadow aspects of themselves and discover who they really are.

Individuals in need of Copaiba often find that vulnerable self-awareness work reveals unresolved pain in hidden recesses of their heart, mind, and body. Many discover they are plagued with feelings of guilt, shame, inadequacy, or unworthiness that have been absorbed from their early environment. These shame-based feelings distort every interaction they have with life. Everything seen through the filter of "less than" creates a perception of the world that is extremely painful and ultimately defeating. Copaiba offers assistance to those caught in lower vibrations of shame, blame, fear, and self-loathing, and other unconsciously internalized emotions. It summons them to begin the unraveling and restoration process necessary for lasting healing and further awareness and insight.

Copaiba invites those who have done something that causes guilt or shame to undergo appropriate remorse and then move on, remembering that forgiveness of the self is also necessary. If not dealt with, these lowest vibrational emotions will drive an individual to rebel or overcompensate. Both are a product of running from their center of truth and existence. Acknowledging the reality of past choices and experiences allows individuals to grow and change in more conscious and clear ways.

Copaiba also invites individuals to come to the Divine for clarity and redefinition. It reminds that the Divine knows them anciently as whole beings—from their earliest childhood wounds to their current limitations. The Divine, as the source and connecting force of everything, possesses the wisdom that transcends mortal perception. Copaiba reassures that mental, emotional, physical, and spiritual limitations are only temporary.

The Divine does not expect individuals to navigate the challenges of life alone or avoid the things they need to experience in life to produce necessary growth and change. Instead, Copaiba teaches that the Divine will reveal the higher message of one's life. It will unveil that they have always been treasured, accepted, valued, worthy of love, and much more. Copaiba imparts that it is only through this divine unveiling that individuals can fully accept the magnificence of what they really are and make peace with the past.

NEGATIVE EMOTIONS: Shameful, guilty, regretful, self-loathing, less than, unworthy, suppressing emotions, rebelling

POSITIVE PROPERTIES: Worthy, self-aware, clarity, forgiven, redefinition of self, purposeful existence

COMPANION OILS: Helichrysum, Frankincense, Black Pepper, Forgive®, HD Clear®, Pink Pepper, Tulsi

SUGGESTED USES:
Aromatic: Inhale from bottle, diffuse, or place drops in hand, rub, and inhale.

Topical: Apply 1-3 drops over heart, sacral chakra (lower stomach), on forehead, crown of head, or back of neck.

Internal: Take 1-2 drops under the tongue, in a capsule, or in water.

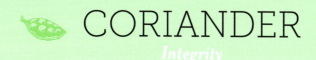

CORIANDER
Integrity

Coriander is the oil of integrity, specifically integrity with oneself. The person in need of Coriander oil may be trapped in a cycle of serving others while neglecting their own needs. They may also have a strong desire to do what is right or correct. Often the mind's perspective of the right way is too limited when seen from only one perspective. Coriander reminds individuals that there is more than one way to do something, and that fitting in often requires betraying the True Self.

Coriander moves the individual from doing things for the acceptance of others to honoring and living from the True Self. There are as many ways of being as there are people in the world. Each soul must learn its own way of living and being. Coriander gives courage to step out of the box and risk being who one really is.

Coriander teaches that each individual is a gift to the world with something unique, which no one else has to offer. Only they can express their uniqueness. Integrity with oneself means living in connection with what one's spirit urges and directs. Coriander helps individuals live from the True Self.

NEGATIVE EMOTIONS: Controlled by others, self-betrayal, drudgery, conforming

POSITIVE PROPERTIES: True to self, inner guidance, integrity, unique

COMPANION OILS: Roman Chamomile, Ginger, Kumquat

SUGGESTED USES:
Aromatic: Inhale from bottle, diffuse, or place drops in hand, rub, and inhale.

Topical: Apply 1-3 drops over solar plexus (upper stomach) or on bottom of feet.

Internal: Take 1-2 drops under the tongue, in a capsule, or in water.

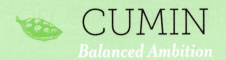

CUMIN
Balanced Ambition

Cumin oil is a balancing force for personal will and ambition. Cumin teaches that while motivation and drive can be powerful catalysts for change, individuals lose integrity when that ambition comes at the expense of others. Often, individuals allow their attachment to a desired outcome to eclipse the needs and feelings of those in their family or social group. They can falsely believe that their enthusiasm for their personal desires or goals make up for inconveniences and insensitivities imposed on others. Cumin addresses this imbalance in relationships, inviting individuals to surrender their unbridled ambition and attachment to outcomes, focusing instead on cooperation and consideration of others.

While cultural norms often teach that success in life is a determinant of happiness, Cumin oil reminds that meaningful relationships have a more direct impact on overall happiness and life satisfaction. This oil warns that when one's drive to reach the top is at the expense of others, they arrive alone.

Cumin also encourages individuals who struggle with a self-centered existence to dig deeper into what is causing these behaviors. Individuals often find the underlying cause may be fear of failure, not being important, not being valued, or not having enough. Cumin eases the anxiousness of these deeper emotional states, encouraging healing from within. It also invites individuals to address the scarcity mindset that drives them to over-impose their will. Additionally, Cumin encourages the positive aspects of zeal that come from feeling secure, respectful, valuable, and energized, without being overbearing. It teaches that healthy zeal comes from knowing why individuals pursue their course and helps them feel confident to accomplish their life mission and goals.

NEGATIVE EMOTIONS: Overly ambitious, insensitive, attached to outcomes, self-centered, fear of failure, scarcity

POSITIVE PROPERTIES: Balanced zeal, considerate, respectful, nonattachment to success, abundant thinking

COMPANION OILS: Oregano, Wild Orange, Lemongrass, Spikenard, Coriander, Basil, Laurel Leaf

SUGGESTED USES:
Aromatic: Inhale from a bottle or diffuse.

Topical: Dilute 1 drop or less with carrier oil and apply over solar plexus (upper stomach) or on bottom of feet. **NOTE**: Use caution when applying topically.

Internal: Take 1-2 drops under the tongue, in a capsule, or in water.

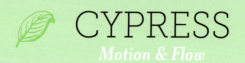

CYPRESS
Motion & Flow

This powerful oil creates energetic flow and emotional catharsis. Stagnant energies are brought into motion through the fluid energy of this oil. Cypress works in the heart and mind, creating flexibility.

Cypress teaches the soul how to let go of the past by moving with the flow of life. This oil is especially indicated for individuals who are mentally or emotionally stuck, stiff, rigid, tense, overstriving, or have perfectionistic tendencies. This hard driving stems from fear and the need to control. The individual tries to force things in life rather than allowing them to unfold naturally.

Cypress encourages individuals to cast aside their worries and let go of control so they can enjoy the thrill that comes from being alive. It reminds individuals that damnation is simply the discontinuation of growth and development, and invites them to step out of the way and allow life to flow freely or without compulsion. Cypress shows how to have perfect trust in the flow of life.

NEGATIVE EMOTIONS: Controlling, fearful, perfectionistic, rigid, stuck, tense

POSITIVE PROPERTIES: Flexible, trusting, flowing with life, adaptable

COMPANION OILS: Wintergreen, Cilantro, Thyme, AromaTouch®, Hinoki, Davana

SUGGESTED USES:
Aromatic: Inhale from bottle, diffuse, or place drops in hand, rub, and inhale.

Topical: Apply 1-3 drops along spine or on bottom of feet.

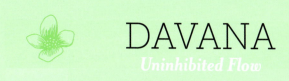

DAVANA
Uninhibited Flow

Davana is a distinctive oil as its aroma is unique to each individual. It changes and adapts to each person's specific chemistry and emotional needs. It is used to treat a wide range of physical ailments and is equally broad in its emotional diversity. Davana is both calming and strengthening. It helps release tension and increase the flow of creative energy. It addresses the fears which stop individuals from feeling the full range of their emotions, inviting them to trust the process of life and allow things to unfold naturally.

This oil assists with a wide range of sacral chakra issues and imbalances. It invites deeper awareness of the ability to connect with the self and with others in more intimate and vulnerable ways. It reveals how much is being held back, kept safe, and suppressed. It helps manifest healthy sexuality and assists individuals in being more comfortable in their own skin. Davana encourages all to embrace the gift of their bodies, get in touch with their sensuality, and allow themselves permission to experience desire.

Davana facilitates reclaiming personal power and belief in the ability to create healthier connections than in the past. It helps individuals to clearly invite what will serve and enhance their life, and repel what weakens them and drains their life force. This oil imbues them with the confidence and courage they need to choose a life full of passion and purpose.

NEGATIVE EMOTIONS: Blocked creativity, fearful, passionless, sexually inhibited, suppressed

POSITIVE PROPERTIES: Creative, trusting, passionate, healthy sexuality, flowing, confident

COMPANION OILS: Jasmine, Neroli, Tangerine, Clove, Cypress, Frankincense, Vetiver, Patchouli, Marjoram

SUGGESTED USES:

Aromatic: Inhale from bottle, diffuse, or place drops in hand, rub, and inhale.

Topical: Dilute 1 drop with carrier oil and apply just below naval or on lower back.

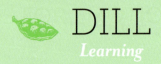

DILL
Learning

Dill supports individuals in learning new things, thinking rationally, and integrating different thoughts into coherent ideas.

This oil is especially helpful for those who feel despondent, bored, or disinterested in the learning process. It supports those who have a difficult time engaging, especially in the classroom. Dill is helpful for those who may feel overwhelmed by too many ideas or by too much stimulus in their environment. Dill can assist individuals to digest and integrate all this information. It supports the left and right brain in working together harmoniously. It can also assist individuals in overcoming mental sluggishness by encouraging awake, alert involvement.

Dill encourages individuals to embrace the many facets of life by engaging in the learning process. It challenges them to become self-motivated learners and to find excitement for discovering new things. It assists individuals in assimilating different thoughts and ideas.

NEGATIVE EMOTIONS: Bored, disinterested, disengaged, overstimulated

POSITIVE PROPERTIES: Engaged, motivated, integrated, mental clarity

COMPANION OILS: Rosemary, Lemon, DigestZen®

SUGGESTED USES:
Aromatic: Inhale from bottle, diffuse, or place drops in hand, rub, and inhale.

Topical: Apply 1-3 drops on back of neck or over solar plexus (upper stomach).

Internal: Take 1-2 drops under the tongue, in a capsule, or in water.

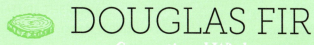

DOUGLAS FIR
Generational Wisdom

Douglas Fir and White Fir share many similar qualities; however Douglas firs live a longer life and would be considered the older and wiser of the two trees. They both address generational issues by inviting individuals to break free from destructive traditions passed down through their families. Douglas Fir assists individuals to live according to their own conscience and values by letting go of harmful patterns. It teaches that each generation can be a gift of new life, new growth, and new beginnings. Similarly, Douglas Fir can also assist with increasing the bond within one's family. It encourages healthy family dynamics where people and meaningful relationships are valued over blind loyalty to traditions.

Additionally, Douglas Fir teaches individuals to learn from and value others' experiences, especially one's family and ancestors. It encourages respect for one's elders and ancestral heritage. Douglas Fir reminds individuals that valuable wisdom can be obtained by learning from the past, especially from individuals who are older, wiser, and more experienced.

NEGATIVE EMOTIONS: Negative generational patterns, burdened by family issues

POSITIVE PROPERTIES: Generational healing, respect for elders, wisdom, learning from the past

COMPANION OILS: Siberian Fir, Petitgrain

SUGGESTED USES:
Aromatic: Inhale from bottle, diffuse, or place drops in hand, rub, and inhale.

Topical: Apply 1-3 drops on base of spine or bottom of feet.

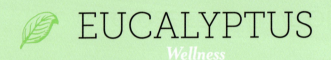

EUCALYPTUS
Wellness

The strong menthol-like aroma of Eucalyptus demonstrates its powerful effect upon the physical and emotional bodies. Eucalyptus oil supports the soul who is constantly facing immune compromising situations. They may be well for a time, only to return to attracting the common afflictions of the season. Eucalyptus teaches that individuals hold unresolved emotional pain in their heart center, and specifically, in their lungs. It invites individuals to respond to their apparent physical susceptibility by also addressing the underlying emotions behind their symptoms.

Eucalyptus addresses a deep emotional or spiritual issue of the need to be unwell or inundated. It reveals patterns of thinking that continually create compromised health. These beliefs may include thoughts such as "I don't deserve to be well," "I am the sort of person who is always getting sick," or "The only way I can get a break is to get sick." Eucalyptus gives individuals courage to face these issues and beliefs. It encourages them to let go of their attachments to being the victim of compromise.

Eucalyptus encourages individuals to take full responsibility for their own health. It bestows trust that one's needs and desires can be met, even if they allow themselves to be well. Eucalyptus teaches how to claim wholeness and health.

NEGATIVE EMOTIONS: Attached to feeling sick or afflicted, clingy, defeated, despairing, desire to escape life or responsibilities, imprisoned, powerless to heal

POSITIVE PROPERTIES: Able to heal, whole, well, liberated, responsible, encouraged

COMPANION OILS: Breathe®^{dōTERRA}, Fennel, Lime, Patchouli, Spikenard

SUGGESTED USES:
Aromatic: Inhale from bottle or diffuse.

Topical: Dilute 2-4 drops with carrier oil and apply over lungs, chest, or throat.

FENNEL

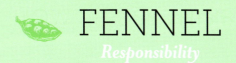

Responsibility

Fennel supports the individual who has a weakened sense of self. The individual may feel defeated by life's responsibilities, having little or no desire to improve their situation. Fennel reignites a passion for life. It encourages the soul to take full ownership and responsibility for its choices. Fennel teaches that life is not too much or too big to handle.

Fennel encourages individuals to live in integrity with themselves, despite the judgments of others. When they have been paralyzed by fear and shame, this oil gets them moving again. Fennel reestablishes a strong connection to the body and the self when there has been weakness or separation.

Fennel also supports an individual in listening to the subtle messages of the body. This is especially important in situations where there has been a loss of connection to the body's natural signals due to emotional eating, severe dieting, eating issues, or drug abuse. Through attunement with the body's actual needs, Fennel curbs cravings for experiences that dull the senses. This oil then supports the individual in hearing the body's signals of hunger, thirst, satiation, or exhaustion. Fennel is also supportive in regaining one's appetite for nourishment, food, and life itself.

NEGATIVE EMOTIONS: Lack of desire, unwilling to take responsibility, shameful, weak sense of self, numb to body signals

POSITIVE PROPERTIES: Responsible, in tune with body, satiated

COMPANION OILS: Ginger, Tangerine, Grapefruit, Patchouli, Blue Tansy, Eucalyptus, Turmeric

SUGGESTED USES:
Aromatic: Inhale from bottle or diffuse.

Topical: Dilute 1-3 drops with carrier oil and apply over entire stomach before or after meals.

Internal: Take 1-2 drops under the tongue, in a capsule, or in water.

FRANKINCENSE
Truth

Frankincense reveals deceptions and false truths. It invites individuals to let go of lower vibrations, lies, deceptions, and negativity. This oil helps create new perspectives based on light and truth. Frankincense recalls to memory spiritual understanding, gifts, wisdom, and knowledge that the soul brought into the world. It is a powerful cleanser of spiritual darkness. Frankincense assists in pulling the "scales of darkness" from the eyes, the barriers from the mind, and the walls from the heart. Through connecting the soul with its inner light, this oil reveals the truth.

Frankincense supports in creating a healthy attachment with one's father. It assists in spiritual awakening and helps individuals feel the love of the Divine. When they have felt abandoned or forgotten, Frankincense reminds them that they are loved and protected. While this oil is incredibly powerful, it is also gentle, like a loving father who nurtures, guides, and protects. Frankincense shields the body and soul from negative influences and assists the soul in its spiritual evolution. Enhancing practices of prayer and meditation, this oil opens spiritual channels that allow an individual to connect to God. Through the light and power of Frankincense, the individual can draw closer to divinity, healthy masculinity, and the grandeur of the True Self.

NEGATIVE EMOTIONS: Abandoned, spiritually disconnected, distant from father, unprotected, spiritual darkness, misaligned

POSITIVE PROPERTIES:
Enlightened, loved, protected, wisdom, discerning, spiritually open, connected to father

COMPANION OILS: Melissa, Manuka, Myrrh, Litsea, Roman Chamomile, Yarrow | Pom

SUGGESTED USES:
Aromatic: Inhale from bottle, diffuse, or place drops in hand, rub, and inhale.

Topical: Apply 1-3 drops on crown of head, forehead, or behind ears.

Environmental: Add several drops into spray bottle and mist around home.

Internal: Take 1-2 drops under the tongue, in a capsule, or in water.

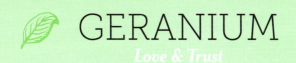

GERANIUM
Love & Trust

Geranium restores confidence in the innate goodness of others and in the world. It facilitates trust, especially when individuals have lost trust in others due to difficult life circumstances. It also assists in reestablishing a strong bond to one's mother and father. When there has been a loss of trust in relationships, Geranium encourages emotional honesty, love, and forgiveness. It fosters receptivity to human love and connection.

Geranium aids in healing the broken heart. It encourages emotional honesty by facilitating the emergence of grief or pain that has been suppressed. Geranium softens anger and assists in healing emotional wounds. It assists in reopening the heart so that love may flow freely. Indeed, Geranium could be called the emotional healer.

Geranium is a gentle oil, perfect for babies and children. It nurtures the inner child and supports in re-parenting this aspect of the self. Individuals who have a difficult time accessing their emotions can be supported by Geranium, as it leads away from the logical mind and into the warmth and nurture of the heart. At its root, Geranium heals the heart, instills unconditional love, and fosters trust.

NEGATIVE EMOTIONS: Abandoned, loss, distrusting, unforgiving, unloving, disheartened, heavyhearted, grieving

POSITIVE PROPERTIES: Emotional healing, empathetic, trusting, forgiving, gentle, loving, tolerant, open

COMPANION OILS: Copaiba, Manuka, Marjoram, Neroli, Ylang Ylang, Rose, Forgive®, Pink Pepper, Bergamot Mint

SUGGESTED USES:
Aromatic: Inhale from bottle or diffuse.

Topical: Dilute 1-3 drops with carrier oil and apply over heart.

Internal: Take 1-2 drops under the tongue, in a capsule, or in water.

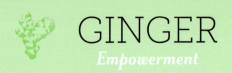

GINGER

Empowerment

Ginger holds no reservations. This oil has a purpose and will fulfill it! Ginger powerfully persuades individuals to be fully present and participate in life. It teaches that to be successful in life, one must be wholly committed to it.

Ginger addresses deep patterns of victim mentality, which is evidenced by feelings of powerlessness, believing everything is outside one's control, refusing to take responsibility for life, or blaming life circumstances on other people or outside influences. Victims feel stuck as they decentralize or disown responsibility and blame others for their misfortunes.

Ginger empowers individuals in taking complete responsibility for their life circumstances. It infuses a warrior-like mentality based on integrity, personal responsibility, and individual choice. Here, individuals see themselves as the creators of their own lives. No longer waiting for outside circumstances to change, they choose their own destiny. The empowered individuals assume full responsibility and accountability for the consequences of their actions or inactions.

NEGATIVE EMOTIONS: Victim mentality, powerless, unwilling to take responsibility, defeated, not present, stuck, blaming others

POSITIVE PROPERTIES: Empowered, committed, capable, purposeful, accountable

COMPANION OILS: Cassia, Fennel, Blue Tansy, Motivate®, Passion®, Spearmint, Star Anise, Turmeric, Laurel Leaf

SUGGESTED USES:

Aromatic: Inhale from bottle or diffuse.

Topical: Dilute 1-2 drops with carrier oil and apply over solar plexus (upper stomach).

Internal: Take 1-2 drops under the tongue, in a capsule, or in water.

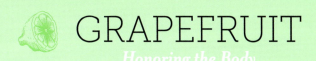

GRAPEFRUIT
Honoring the Body

Grapefruit teaches true respect and appreciation for one's physical body. It supports individuals who struggle to honor their body and are caught in patterns of mistreatment. These forms of abuse may include severe dieting, judging one's body weight or type, and abusing the body through negligent behavior or violence. These acts are often motivated by hate and disgust buried within the psyche, which gets directed toward the physical body. Though individuals may obsess over how they look, deep down they never feel they look good enough. There is a dissatisfaction that persists.

Grapefruit oil is often misused in overly strict dietary and weight-loss programs. The reason this oil helps curb emotional eating is because it encourages a positive relationship with one's body based on love, tolerance, and acceptance. Grapefruit encourages integrity by respecting one's physical needs. This oil assists individuals in listening to their true physical needs and impulses. It also assists them in taking responsibility for what they feel. Grapefruit teaches that no amount of food can fill a hole in the heart—only love can do that. As individuals take ownership of their feelings and get the help they need in addressing them, they no longer have a need to hide their feelings behind food, body abuse, strict regimens, eating issues, or other forms of obsession.

NEGATIVE EMOTIONS: Body shame, obsession with food or dieting, eating issues, distorted self-image, hiding

POSITIVE PROPERTIES: Respectful of physical needs, body acceptance, nourished, healthy relationship with food

COMPANION OILS: Patchouli, Bergamot, Slim & Sassy®, Fennel, Beautiful, Citrus Bloom®

SUGGESTED USES:
Aromatic: Inhale from bottle, diffuse, or place drops in hand, rub, and inhale.
Topical: Apply 1-3 drops on wrists or over entire stomach.
Internal: Take 1-2 drops under the tongue, in a capsule, or in water.

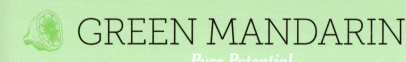

GREEN MANDARIN
Pure Potential

Green Mandarin, the unripe fruit of the mandarin tree, shares similar characteristics with its ripe counterpart. It is an excellent tonic to aid individuals in returning to childhood delight and simplicity. Green Mandarin's bright and cheerful aroma helps all to remember the budding excitement they once felt about life. In adulthood, individuals often feel trapped or limited by their own belief systems. This oil reminds individuals that they have direct access to pure potential and boundless opportunities. It encourages all to experience joy in the journey and to never stop becoming.

When individual are feeling weighed down by emotional scars, self-doubt, fear, or failure, Green Mandarin prompts them to harken back to a time before they were encumbered by this baggage. It reminds them to reconnect to their inner child whose heart was open and fearless. It reassures that fear is temporary and abundant possibilities await those who dare to dream. Green Mandarin reminds that wonder and hope are food for the soul and imparts its exuberance for fully living life.

NEGATIVE EMOTIONS: Limited, trapped, fearful, doubtful, burdened, encumbered

POSITIVE PROPERTIES: Excited, wonder, hopeful, fearless, innocent, delighted

COMPANION OILS: Red Mandarin, Lime, Tangerine, Lemon, Helichrysum, Sunny Citrus, Elevation

SUGGESTED USES:
Aromatic: Inhale from bottle, diffuse, or place drops in hand, rub, and inhale.

Topical: Dilute 1-3 drops with carrier oil and apply around navel over heart, and on wrists.

Internal: Take 1-2 drops under the tongue, in a capsule, or in water.

HELICHRYSUM
Emotional Pain

Helichrysum is an amazing healer of emotional pain. It aids the walking wounded—those with a history of difficult life circumstances, trauma, self-destruction, loss, or abuse. These individuals need the powerful spiritual support that Helichrysum offers. It gives strength and endurance to the wounded soul who must keep on living, despite past difficulties. This oil restores confidence in life and in the self, giving individuals strength to carry on. Helichrysum has a powerful relationship with the light of the sun. It imbues joy, fervor, and hope for living. Helichrysum takes hurt souls by the hand, guiding them through life's difficulties. If individuals can persevere, this oil can take them into new heights of spiritual consciousness. Helichrysum offers hope that their emotional wounds can be healed.

Following this spiritual healing and transformation, Helichrysum can teach individuals to have gratitude for their trials. It helps them to see that if they had not been wounded, they would not have sought healing that resulted in a spiritual rebirth. Just as the phoenix dies and rises from its ashes, so might one be raised from turmoil. Helichrysum lends its warrior spirit so that all may face adversities with courage and determination. It brings hope to the most discouraged of souls and life to those in need of rebirth.

NEGATIVE EMOTIONS: Intense emotional pain, anguish, or trauma; hopeless, despairing, wounded

POSITIVE PROPERTIES: Healing, courageous, hopeful, transforming, persevering, determined

COMPANION OILS: Hope®, Deep Blue®, Ginger, Wintergreen, Lime, Siberian Fir, Peppermint, Bergamot Mint

SUGGESTED USES:
Aromatic: Inhale from bottle, diffuse, or place drops in hand, rub, and inhale.

Topical: Apply 1-3 drops over heart or wherever pain is experienced.

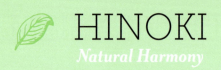

HINOKI
Natural Harmony

Hinoki oil, from the Japanese cypress tree, is relaxing and slightly sedative in nature. Its properties impart a sense of calm and order, similar to walking in a Japanese garden, which is helpful in times of stress and overstimulation. Hinoki soothes individuals when they are feeling hurried, constricted, rigid, or tense.

Hinoki also assists individuals in removing the disorder and disharmony which may have built up within their lives. It creates an energetic fluidity that allows the movement and ultimate release of what is creating the disorder. Hinoki holds a solemn respect for the natural order and universal flow. Without force or haste, it leads individuals into the necessary work of becoming balanced and harmonious once more. It holds an energetic place of being honorable and true that is impervious to outside degradation or influence. In this way, Hinoki teaches individuals how to be more harmonious within their surroundings and less affected by the turbulence of life.

The scent of Hinoki invokes a sacred calm and is excellent for diffusing in places of quiet meditation or religious worship.

NEGATIVE EMOTIONS: Disharmonious, hurried, tense, stressed, disorganized, energetically blocked, unstable

POSITIVE PROPERTIES: Harmonious, calm, ordered, relaxed, respectful, balanced, honorable

COMPANION OILS: Cypress, Sandalwood, Vetiver, Arborvitae, Magnolia

SUGGESTED USES:
Aromatic: Inhale from bottle, diffuse, or place drops in hand, rub, and inhale.

Topical: Apply 1-3 drops on temples, back of neck, and along spine.

*Environmenta*l: Add several drops into spray bottle and mist around home.

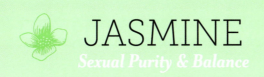

JASMINE
Sexual Purity & Balance

Jasmine nurtures healthy sexuality and helps to balance sexual forces. It may also arouse dormant passions, assisting individuals to regain interest in the sexual experience. Jasmine cultivates positive experiences within intimate relationships by encouraging the purification of unhealthy sexual intentions and motivations. It asks individuals to honor and respect themselves and others.

Jasmine encourages the release of sexual suppression or resistance due to traumatic experiences. Through its gentle, purifying nature, Jasmine brings forward unresolved sexual experiences and facilitates the healing process. Traumatic experiences can distort one's relationship with sexuality. Jasmine can assist both kinds of common compensations: those who fear, repel, or resist the sexual experience, as well as those who obsess over or are fixated on sexuality. It is balancing for individuals who use sex to fill a desperate need for love and approval, as well as individuals who resist sexual intimacy.

Jasmine supports the resolution of sexual issues, encourages safety within intimate relationships, and invites only the purest intentions to the sexual experience.

NEGATIVE EMOTIONS: Unresolved sexual issues, sexual repression or sexual fixation

POSITIVE PROPERTIES: Healthy sexuality, pure intentions, innocent, healing, self-acceptance, intimate, trusting, safe

COMPANION OILS: Cinnamon, Neroli, Davana

SUGGESTED USES:
Aromatic: Inhale from bottle, diffuse, or place drops in hand, rub, and inhale.

Topical: Apply 1-2 drops over sacral chakra (lower stomach), lower back, or behind ears.

JUNIPER BERRY
Night

Juniper Berry assists those who fear the dark or unknown aspects of themselves. It helps individuals to understand that those things they fear are intended to be their teachers. Instead of hiding from what they do not understand, Juniper Berry encourages individuals to learn the lesson and face their fear. These fears often live within the unexplored areas of the self. Juniper Berry acts as a catalyst by helping individuals access and address those fears and issues which have long been avoided.

Dreams contain nighttime communications. Even nightmares can reveal unresolved fears and issues. Juniper Berry offers courage and energetic protection in the nighttime. It encourages an honest assessment of the information being communicated from within. As individuals reconcile with their fears and other hidden aspects of themselves, they experience greater wholeness. Juniper Berry helps restore the balance between light and dark, conscious and subconscious, day and night. It acts as a guide on the path toward wholeness. Juniper Berry teaches that there is truly nothing to fear when one acknowledges and accepts all aspects of the self.

NEGATIVE EMOTIONS: Irrationally fearful, recurrent nightmares, disrupted sleep, avoiding

POSITIVE PROPERTIES: Protected, peaceful dreaming, courageous, self-aware

COMPANION OILS: Black Pepper, Clary Sage, On Guard®, Vetiver

SUGGESTED USES:
Aromatic: Inhale from bottle, diffuse, or place drops in hand, rub, and inhale before bed.

Topical: Apply 1 drop on forehead or behind ears before bed.

Environmental: Add several drops into spray bottle and mist around bedroom.

Internal: Take 1-2 drops under the tongue, in a capsule, or in water.

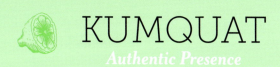

KUMQUAT
Authentic Presence

Kumquats are unique in the citrus family with the sweetest part of the fruit contained on the outside, in the peel. The complexity of complementary flavors lies within. As such, Kumquat oil addresses preoccupation with a cheerful external disposition that masks anxiousness, self-doubt, pain, and unease hidden within.

Individuals in need of Kumquat oil tend to judge and push down feelings deemed as unacceptable or unwanted. Often they have been taught to repress feelings in order to be accepted. These personalities appear happy, enthusiastic, popular, and seemingly at peace in the world while their inner torment is meticulously guarded and hidden from view. However, this denial, avoidance of emotional pain, and fear of negative emotions can lead to destructive coping strategies and passive aggressiveness in order to continue keeping up the chosen facade.

Kumquat oil instructs that true happiness comes only through real, honest, and unstudied living. It reminds that people are a complement of good and bad, sweet and sour. Individuals must embrace their multifaceted humanness and anchor their identity in the truth in order to live authentically. Kumquat invites all to shift their focus away from outward behaviors or pretenses—which others may validate—and instead begin the quiet, consistent, and unseen journey to inner alignment, contentment, and healing.

NEGATIVE EMOTIONS: Superficial, facade of cheerfulness, hiding, inauthentic, repressed feelings, passive aggressive

POSITIVE PROPERTIES: Unstudied, authentic, real, honest, sincere, unpretentious, aligned

COMPANION OILS: Black Pepper, Coriander, Lavender, Pink Pepper

SUGGESTED USES:
Aromatic: Inhale from bottle, diffuse, or place drops in hand, rub, and inhale
Topical: Apply 1-3 drops over throat, stomach, or on forehead.
Internal: Take 1-2 drops under the tongue, in a capsule, or in water.

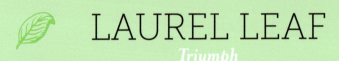

LAUREL LEAF
Triumph

Laurel leaf bolsters one's confidence in the ability to overcome. When individuals are feeling suppressed by their self-doubt, belief deficit, or fear of failure, Laurel imparts an energetic vote of confidence. It teaches that setbacks are the very best teachers, and all who discover their magnificence do so only after they have persevered through numerous failures. Laurel teaches that challenging experiences carve out enough capacity to receive one's eventual triumph.

Laurel works deeply within the individuals to help heal the issues causing them to unconsciously engage in self-sabotage. It shines a light on the parts of them that don't believe they are worthy of good things or wonderful experiences. This oil helps them understand that there is no security in staying small and unnoticed. Laurel teaches them to realize they have more ability than they once believed and encourages them to not settle for less than what they dream of.

Laurel helps individuals grow, expand, and engage in long-term character development. It reminds of the commitment required in lifelong achievement. It is an ally for those who are ready to overcome their fear of success and step into their brilliance. Laurel's energy inspires all to choose greatness and rise up to personal victory.

NEGATIVE EMOTIONS: Fear of failure, fear of success, self-sabotage, self-doubt, unworthy, hiding

POSITIVE PROPERTIES: Triumphant, confident, belief, perseverance, capable, overcoming, victorious

COMPANION OILS: Blue Tansy, Cassia, Cumin, Ginger, Litsea, Spearmint, Turmeric, Adaptiv, Motivate, Passion

SUGGESTED USES:

Aromatic: Inhale from bottle, diffuse, or place drops in hand, rub, and inhale.

Topical: Dilute 1-2 drops with carrier oil and apply over solar plexus (upper stomach), or on bottom of feet.

Environmental: Add several drops into spray bottle and mist around bedroom.

Internal: Take 1-2 drops under the tongue, in a capsule, or in water.

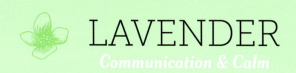

LAVENDER

Communication & Calm

Lavender aids verbal expression and calm the mind. Specifically, it calms the insecurities that are felt when one risks their true thoughts and feelings. Lavender addresses a deep fear of being seen and heard. Individuals in need of Lavender hide within, blocking their true self-expression. While they may be going through the motions of outward expression, they're actually holding back their innermost thoughts and feelings. The expression is not connected to the heart or soul.

Lavender supports individuals in releasing the tension and constriction that stems from withheld expression. This bottleneck in communication can result in worried and racing thoughts, anxiousness, and sleep disruption. Due to past experiences, they may feel unsafe or fearful of expressing themselves because of potential rejection. Often they don't allow themselves space to get in touch with all they truly think and feel. Their true voice is therefore trapped within and goes unexpressed. Strong feelings of being unlovable, unimportant, or unheard can accompany this condition.

Lavender encourages emotional honesty and insists that individuals speak their innermost thoughts and desires. As they learn to communicate their deepest thoughts and feelings, they are liberated from their self-inflicted prison. It is through open and honest communication that individuals have the potential to experience unconditional love, acceptance, and peace of mind. Through Lavender's courageous spirit, all are free to share their True Self with others.

NEGATIVE EMOTIONS: Blocked communication, fear of rejection, constricted, tense, racing thoughts, emotional dishonesty, hiding, fear of self-disclosure, insecure; feeling unseen, unheard, or unloved

POSITIVE PROPERTIES: Open communication, calm, expressive, emotionally honest, self-aware, peace of mind

COMPANION OILS: Spearmint, Serenity®, Citrus Bloom®, Bergamot Mint

SUGGESTED USES:

Aromatic: Inhale from bottle, diffuse, or place drops in hand, rub, and inhale.

Topical: Apply 1-3 drops over throat, on temples, or back of neck.

Internal: Take 1-2 drops under the tongue, in a capsule, or in water.

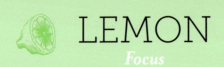

LEMON

Focus

The delightful citrusy aroma of Lemon oil engages the mind and aids concentration. While Lemon supports the emotional body, its major effects are experienced in the mental field. The crisp scent of Lemon oil improves one's ability to focus. Lemon is a wonderful aid for children struggling with school. It teaches individuals to be mentally present by focusing on one thing at a time. Lemon dispels confusion and bestows clarity. It counterbalances mental fatigue due to too much studying or reading. Lemon restores energy, mental flexibility, and the drive to complete a project.

Lemon is especially helpful in cases of learning issues. Whether an individual has a difficult time concentrating or feels incapable of learning, Lemon clears self-judgments such as "I'm dumb" or "I'm not a good student." Lemon calms fears and insecurities while restoring confidence in the self. Emotionally, Lemon inspires a natural playfulness and buoyancy in the heart. It assists in releasing feelings of despair and hopelessness by restoring feelings of joy and happiness. Lemon inspires joyful involvement in the present moment by infusing the soul with energy, confidence, and alertness.

NEGATIVE EMOTIONS: Confused, unable to focus, mentally fatigued, lacking joy and energy, learning issues, guilty, disengaged

POSITIVE PROPERTIES: Focused, energized, mental clarity, alert, rational, joyful

COMPANION OILS: Rosemary, Dill, Peppermint, Sunny Citrus, InTune®, Green Mandarin, Lemon Myrtle, Harvest Spice, Island Mint®

SUGGESTED USES:

Aromatic: Inhale from bottle or diffuse before mental exertion or during work or study.

Topical: Dilute 1-3 drops with carrier oil and apply on wrists and temples.

Internal: Take 1-2 drops under the tongue, in a capsule, or in water.

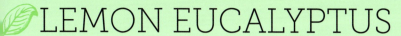

LEMON EUCALYPTUS
Protected Space

Lemon Eucalyptus creates protected space around individuals. This is especially helpful when they are feeling overly exposed to natural elements or energetic forces. Feeling self-contained is an energetic need and a human right. Individuals become disoriented and less effective when they have been too open and exposed to external energies for too long. Lemon Eucalyptus helps individuals recognize when they need to create more effective boundaries and maintain their personal space.

Lemon Eucalyptus is a powerful cleanser of energetic debris. In this way it has the unique ability to lessen the impact of challenging energies and circumstances. It assists individuals in purifying their environment, which frees up mental and spiritual resources. Lemon Eucalyptus offers reinforcement and resolve when individuals need to more independently navigate their lives.

NEGATIVE EMOTIONS: Exposed, unprotected, enmeshed, poor boundaries, energetically weakened

POSITIVE PROPERTIES: Self-contained, reinforced, protected, clear boundaries

COMPANION OILS: TerraShield®, Tea Tree, Lemongrass, On Guard®, Purify, Citronella

SUGGESTED USES:
Aromatic: Inhale from bottle, diffuse, or place drops in hand, rub, and inhale.

Topical: Dilute 1-2 drops with carrier oil and apply on bottom of feet.

Environmental: Add several drops into spray bottle and mist around home.

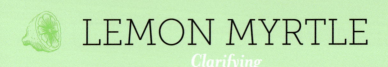

LEMON MYRTLE

Clarifying

Lemon Myrtle is a bright, fresh, and uplifting aroma. It's extremely effective in cutting through the prevalent modern states of mental fogginess, dull senses, and living on autopilot. The nature of the modern lifestyle leads to overstimulation through the constant barrage of new information and experiences. Often individuals react by mentally shutting down or getting lost in circling and unproductive thoughts. Lemon Myrtle can help calm and redirect erratic thoughts and invigorate the mind.

Lemon Myrtle assists individuals in releasing accumulated toxicity acquired through unconscious absorption of negative group thought and lower energetic vibrations. If individuals begin to exhibit signs that they are not thinking clearly or making rational decisions, this oil acts as a purgative to clear and dispel negative influences and unwelcome intrusions. It is a powerful cleanser which brings a sense of relief and the freedom for individuals to think for themselves again.

Lemon Myrtle promotes positive, clear thinking. It also helps with clarifying the mind and will. It provides a powerful lift that revitalizes the energy system enabling all to intentionally choose the vibrational energy to which they attune.

NEGATIVE EMOTIONS: Mental fog, dulled senses, overstimulated, erratic, compulsive, absorbing negative energy, easily influenced, emotionally toxic, confused

POSITIVE PROPERTIES: Clarity, intentional, calm, rational, mentally invigorated, free

COMPANION OILS: Tea Tree, Lemon, Lemongrass, Purify

SUGGESTED USES:
Aromatic: Inhale from bottle or diffuse.
Topical: Dilute 1 drop with carrier oil and apply on bottom of feet. **NOTE:** Use caution when applying topically.
Environmental: Add several drops into spray bottle and mist around home.
Internal: Take 1-2 drops under the tongue, in a capsule, or in water.

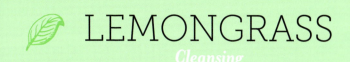

LEMONGRASS
Cleansing

Lemongrass is a powerful cleanser of energy. It dispels feelings of despondency, despair, and lethargy. Lemongrass assists individuals in entering a healing mode or cleansing state. In this state, one easily lets go of old, limiting beliefs, toxic energies, and negativity. Lemongrass teaches individuals to move forward without hesitation. It asks them to commit to a healing path where change is a regular occurrence.

Lemongrass can also be a powerful tool in cleansing the energy within a house, room, or work space. It encourages individuals with hoarding tendencies to courageously let go of everything they no longer need.

Lemongrass also clears negative energy from the brow chakra or spiritual eyes. As individuals let go of past issues and stagnant energy, they have an increased ability to see situations with greater clarity. It supports individuals' energy in flowing freely and smoothly. Lemongrass has a powerful mission to assist in cleansing physically, emotionally, and spiritually.

NEGATIVE EMOTIONS: Toxic or negative energy, despairing, holding on to the past, hoarding, darkness, spiritual blindness

POSITIVE PROPERTIES: Spiritual clarity, cleansing, nonattachment, simplicity, discerning, releasing the unneeded

COMPANION OILS: Clary Sage, Sandalwood, Oregano, Thyme, Purify, Lemon Myrtle

SUGGESTED USES:
Aromatic: Inhale from bottle or diffuse.

Topical: Dilute 1-2 drops with carrier oil and apply on bottom of feet.

Environmental: Add several drops into spray bottle and mist around home.

Internal: Take 1-2 drops under the tongue, in a capsule, or in water.

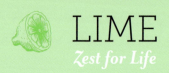

LIME
Zest for Life

Lime imbues the soul with a zest for life. When individuals have been weighed down by discouragement or grief, Lime elevates them above the mire. It instills courage and cheer in the heart and reminds them to be grateful for the gift of life.

Lime cleanses the heart, especially when there has been an accumulation of emotional toxins due to avoidance or repression. This oil revitalizes the heart space, giving room for light and joy. It clears discouragement and thoughts and feelings related to a loss of will to live. Lime shines light on the inner motives hidden in the heart and encourages emotional honesty.

Lime can also assist individuals who have overly developed their intellectual capacities but have neglected to develop themselves emotionally. This oil encourages balance between the heart and mind. It clears congestion from the heart region, assisting individuals in feeling safe and at home in their heart. Lime dispels apathy and resignation, and instills hope, joy, courage, and the determination to face all of life's challenges.

NEGATIVE EMOTIONS: Apathetic, resigned, grieving, loss of will to live, discouraged

POSITIVE PROPERTIES: Courageous, emotionally honest, engaged, revitalized, determined, grateful for life

COMPANION OILS: Tangerine, Melissa, Spikenard, Sunny Citrus, Elevation, Green Mandarin, Harvest Spice, Island Mint®

SUGGESTED USES:
Aromatic: Inhale from bottle or diffuse.

Topical: Dilute 1-3 drops with carrier oil and apply over chest.

Internal: Take 1-2 drops under the tongue, in a capsule, or in water.

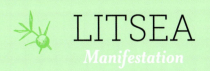

LITSEA
Manifestation

Litsea is a powerful mobilizer of the will. It is especially helpful in encouraging individuals to follow through on their inspiration and promptings. Generally, individuals have many intuitive moments when their mind is open and connected to their higher consciousness. In this receptive state, information and energy flow freely. However, these inspirations are often shut down or discarded as individuals judge, criticize, and stifle the light they receive. Litsea invites all to have the confidence to act on the information given and to trust in wisdom that may be beyond current understanding.

Litsea instills courage to face the fear that comes immediately after inspiration. It reminds individuals that it takes a leap of faith into the unknown in order to manifest what has been previously unrealized. This oil also teaches that one must learn to trust the inner voice and rise above fear of rejection, being misunderstood, or the need for external confirmation.

Litsea invites individuals to recognize what clouds and distracts their internal clarity and to make the required changes to live in greater alignment. It acts as a catalyst for living in accordance with one's higher purpose and internal compass and helps individuals to get out of their own way. As such, Litsea assists in the manifestation of infinite possibilities.

NEGATIVE EMOTIONS: Self-doubt and criticism, stifled, fear of rejection, relying on external confirmation, distracted, blocked, limited

POSITIVE PROPERTIES: Inspired, intuitive, aligned, receptive, manifesting, trusting of inner voice, clarity, open to possibilities

COMPANION OILS: Blue Tansy, Clary Sage, Melissa, Lemongrass, Turmeric, Laurel Leaf

SUGGESTED USES:
Aromatic: Inhale from bottle or diffuse.
Topical: Dilute 1-3 drops with carrier oil and apply on forehead, temples, or back of neck.
Internal: Take 1-2 drops under the tongue, in a capsule, or in water.

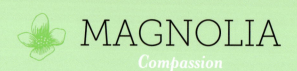

MAGNOLIA

Compassion

Magnolia connects people with the energy of the Divine Matriarch. This feminine spiritual source expects individuals to treat one another with mercy and compassion. Magnolia creates a tender place within the heart to learn important lessons about human interconnectedness and how to live in love and harmony. It also assists in illuminating the distance between individuals and dispels whatever may be clouding the ability to see other human beings with relatable needs, desires, and pains. It encourages all individuals on a profoundly spiritual level to interact without causing pain or suffering, and to refrain from seeing others as somehow less than oneself.

The inviting sweetness of Magnolia draws the senses in with gentle, pure, maternal nurturing that facilitates deep healing and soul-level change. Once individuals feel safe and loved, they will naturally see where they are withholding compassion from themselves and from those around them. Magnolia inspires all to engage with their fellow sojourners in this life with greater and greater empathy. It mirrors back to each individual the shared humanity reflected in another's eyes and reminds that each soul is equally deserving of kindness and respect. Magnolia reveals the essential bonds shared between all people. When individuals view themselves as separate from others, they begin to lose the thread that weaves humanity together and to disregard the outcomes of the people they have detached themselves from. Magnolia facilitates a divine healing energy bringing the world a remedy for these soul sicknesses.

Magnolia inspires the willingness to see the divine beauty within each soul. It teaches that each individual shares a responsibility to discover the gaps in their connection to others, to clear the encumbered perceptions obscuring truth, and to turn to the Divine to heal those cold, confused, or barren places within their understanding. Magnolia offers a true haven of refuge and reflection and inspires deep, transformative thought. Magnolia is a tonic for those who feel separated from the Divine Feminine and desperately need the lost teachings of a loving parent to guide them on the path to greater happiness, progress, and unity.

NEGATIVE EMOTIONS: Disconnected, numb, lonely, isolated, withdrawn, justifying, unsympathetic, unkind

POSITIVE PROPERTIES: Connected, compassionate, interconnected, unified, thoughtful, insightful, perceptive, respectful, kind

COMPANION OILS: Myrrh, Rose, Cedarwood, Marjoram, Manuka, Arborvitae, Citrus Bloom®, Tulsi

SUGGESTED USES:
Aromatic: Inhale from bottle or place a few drops in hand, rub, and inhale.

Topical: Apply to center of chest (heart center) or on crown of head.

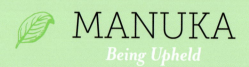

MANUKA

Being Upheld

Manuka is a powerful plant given as a gift to the earth to heal and bless humanity. It carries a unique energy signature that raises the vibration of those who come in contact with it. The purposes of Manuka are multifaceted, each part adding its mission to its divine whole. Manuka's primary message is to remind individuals that they are known by the Divine. Like every flower and sparrow, each person is known, loved, and cared for. Manuka invites the heart to open to the gifts bestowed daily in abundance and to live in states of gratitude and wonder.

Manuka also offers powerful healing energy to bind up wounds, soothe troubled hearts, and nurture souls back into a state of centeredness. Its special alchemy transforms lower states of consciousness into higher vibrations and awareness. It facilitates a connection between heaven and earth, and encourages access to that sacred space where individuals can rest and simply be upheld by the Divine.

Manuka offers energetic safety and shielding from the intense problems all around that individuals feel powerless to change. Once individuals surrender the weights and burdens they carry, they are free to connect to the overflowing divine goodness waiting for them. Manuka helps individuals understand they occupy a unique space in the universe, there is always enough for them, and they will be taken care of. It reminds that even though there are things to grieve, divine love will return beauty for ashes.

NEGATIVE EMOTIONS: Wounded, abandoned, forsaken, suffering, disconnected, unsafe, powerless, burdened, grieving

POSITIVE PROPERTIES: Soothed, comforted, healing, loved, cared for, upheld, and known by the Divine, grateful, transcendence

COMPANION OILS: Rose, Melissa, Frankincense, Spikenard, Arborvitae, Myrrh, Copaiba, Breathe®, Magnolia

SUGGESTED USES:
Aromatic: Inhale from bottle, diffuse, or place drops in hand, rub, and inhale.

Topical: Apply 1-3 drops over heart, on crown of head, forehead, or base of spine.

Environmental: Add several drops into spray bottle and mist around body or home.

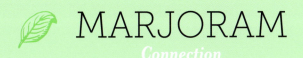

MARJORAM

Connection

Marjoram aids those who are unable to trust others or form meaningful relationships. This inability to trust often stems from harsh life experiences. These individuals develop a fear of close connection in relationships. They may tend toward reclusive behaviors, protecting themselves even further by abstaining from social interactions. They may also protect themselves by unconsciously sabotaging long-term relationships.

Marjoram shows the barriers individuals have formed to protect themselves from others. It reveals patterns of aloofness, distancing oneself from other people, or being cold. Those in need of Marjoram oil most likely use these protective coping strategies unintentionally. Deep down, they desire the intimate connection they subconsciously sabotage.

Marjoram teaches that trust is the basis for all relationships. It assists individuals in increasing their warmth and trust in social situations. Marjoram softens the heart and heals past wounds. It kindles the fires of trust in relationships so that one may fully blossom. When individuals feel safe and loved, they express their authenticity more freely. Marjoram restores trust and openness so that true bonds of love may be formed in friendships and relationships.

NEGATIVE EMOTIONS: Distrusting, emotionally aloof or distant, overly protective, emotionally isolated, reclusive, fear of rejection, self-sabotage

POSITIVE PROPERTIES: Emotionally open and connected, close relationships, softhearted, loving, trusting

COMPANION OILS: Cedarwood, Neroli, Geranium, Magnolia

SUGGESTED USES:
Aromatic: Inhale from bottle, diffuse, or place drops in hand, rub, and inhale.

Topical: Apply 1-3 drops over heart and chest.

Internal: Take 1-2 drops under the tongue, in a capsule, or in water.

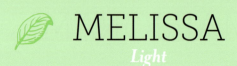

MELISSA
Light

Melissa oil awakens the soul to truth and light. It reminds individuals of who they truly are and why they came to this earth. Melissa invites one to release everything and anything that holds them back from reaching their fullest potential.

Melissa assists individuals in receiving spiritual guidance by reconnecting them with their inner voice. It uplifts the soul by preparing one to ascend. When individuals feel too weighed down by the burdens of life, Melissa encourages them to keep going. It gives strength and vitality to the innermost recesses of the heart and soul. This oil invites all to participate in higher realms of living and dreaming. As they stay connected to spiritual sources, they feel lightness in their being and brightness in their core. Melissa reminds everyone that each individual has a spark of divinity within them, and with love and attention, the spark will grow. This oil fuels that spark of energy, igniting an individual's True Self. Melissa assists them in shedding everything that is not in harmony with their inner light.

Melissa's enthusiasm is contagious. Through the intense light and vibration this oil has to offer, individuals may feel they cannot help but let go of feelings of darkness, despair, and other low vibrations that are holding them down. It teaches the joy of living.

NEGATIVE EMOTIONS: Despairing, hopeless, darkness, burdened, loss of will to live, overwhelmed

POSITIVE PROPERTIES: Enlightened, joyful, energized, integrity, spiritually connected, contagious enthusiasm, liberated, optimistic

COMPANION OILS: Frankincense, Copaiba, Peppermint, Tangerine, Lime, Yarrow | Pom, Tulsi

SUGGESTED USES:

Aromatic: Inhale from bottle, diffuse, or place drops in hand, rub, and inhale.

Topical: Apply 1-2 drops on forehead or ears. Apply 1 drop to pad of thumb then press against roof of mouth, for 30 seconds.

Internal: Take 1-2 drops under the tongue, in a capsule, or in water.

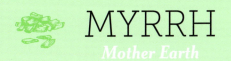

MYRRH
Mother Earth

Myrrh oil nurtures the soul's relationship with its maternal mother and with the earth. This oil supports individuals who have had disturbances with the mother-child bond. Whether it's a division between the child and the biological mother or Mother Earth herself, Myrrh can help bridge the gap and heal the disturbance. This division or lack of attachment may be related to adoption, birth trauma, malnourishment, experiences of abandonment, or other childhood issues. Myrrh helps the soul to feel the love and nurturing presence of a mother. Similar to the nutrient-rich colostrum found in a mother's milk, Myrrh oil inoculates individuals from the emotionally adverse and harmful effects of the world. Like the warmth of a mother's love for her child, Myrrh assists individuals in feeling safe and secure.

When the mother-child bond has been disrupted, the soul may lose its childlike ability to trust. Feelings of trust are replaced with feelings of fear and a belief that the world is unsafe. Myrrh assists individuals in letting go of fear. Through reestablishing a healthy connection to the earth and to one's own mother, Myrrh rekindles trust within the soul. As the individual learns to once again live in trust, confidence in the goodness of life returns and the soul feels safe and more at home.

NEGATIVE EMOTIONS: Disrupted maternal connection, distrusting, neglected, unsafe in the world, malnourished

POSITIVE PROPERTIES: Safe in the world, healthy attachments, trusting, bonding, maternal connection, nurtured, loved, secure, grounded

COMPANION OILS: Rose, Frankincense, Manuka, ClaryCalm®, Magnolia, Star Anise

SUGGESTED USES:
Aromatic: Inhale from bottle, diffuse, or place drops in hand, rub, and inhale.

Topical: Apply 1-3 drops over heart, chest, around navel, or on bottom of feet.

Internal: Take 1-2 drops under the tongue, in a capsule, or in water.

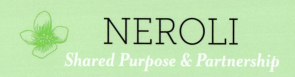

NEROLI
Shared Purpose & Partnership

Neroli is a unifying and stabilizing oil. It is particularly helpful for calming troubled hearts in relationship conflict. Its influence promotes harmony in the changing dynamics of long-term relationships. Ongoing partnerships require acceptance and growth. Over time, perceived weaknesses in others come into full view, and, as a result, individuals can grow bitter, frustrated, unsympathetic, and create emotional distance from people they once loved and cherished. If left unchecked, these feelings can grow into dysfunctional and destructive thoughts and behaviors. Perceived stagnation in a relationship can cause despair and apathy, and feed a desire to blame, punish, or escape. Alternatively, Neroli invites individuals to develop the character traits of fidelity, empathy, patience, forgiveness, and resilience to ease these relationship challenges.

Neroli assists with the positive evolution of sexual intimacy between individuals who have been together long enough to experience significant contrasts in their sexual relationship. It symbolizes the fleeting beauty of spring blossoms and honors the long-lasting creation cycle in the life of the tree. Neroli aids in realizing deeper states of connection in intimate moments. It also encourages individuals to address the emotional barriers that impede healthy sexual expression and connection. Neroli gently reminds that sexual unity is a key aspect of relationship happiness, and to take the time to nurture this process.

Neroli teaches that unity blossoms from adaptation, cooperation, tolerance, perseverance, and kindness. It encourages active acceptance and supportive space for the chosen partner. Neroli invites individuals to attune their focus to the beautiful tapestry that is created as two lives intertwine to share purpose and find meaning.

NEGATIVE EMOTIONS: Conflicted, restless, impatient, bitter, frustrated, unsympathetic, disloyal, dispassionate, sexual inhibition, aloof, unkind, stagnant, blaming, escapism

POSITIVE PROPERTIES: Patient, empathetic, kind, tolerant, fidelity, calm, intimate, sexual desire, resilient, cooperative, committed

COMPANION OILS: Geranium, Jasmine, Cinnamon, Whisper®, Marjoram, Spikenard, ClaryCalm®, Davana

SUGGESTED USES:

Aromatic: Inhale from bottle, diffuse, or place drops in hand, rub, and inhale.

Topical: Apply 1-3 drops over heart, sacral chakra (lower stomach), throat, or behind ears.

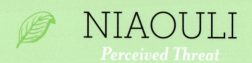

NIAOULI
Perceived Threat

Niaouli assists individuals when they are feeling threatened and self-protective. Individuals oftentimes react aggressively when other's opinions and choices offend their sense of order, justice, or right. This oil assists in recalibrating emotional responses when one has become irritated, irrational, or inflamed by the decisions of others. It helps individuals recognize that perceived threats are manifestations of their own beliefs and biases, and that ideological differences do not represent actual harm. It reminds individuals that they have the power to choose rational and kind responses in each situation they find themselves in.

Niaouli is an excellent ally in working with the ego. It teaches that challenges to an individual's self-construct reveal the work they have yet to do. This oil cuts through the justification for their combative choices and preemptive strikes against others. It helps individuals resist the impulse to make others wrong. It reveals that the true cause of defensiveness is a sense of powerlessness that can be addressed and healed.

Niaouli reveals the false boundaries individuals have set for others in order to feel safe. This oil's message is that emotional safety comes, not from contending with the outside world, but from clearing out the toxicity and discord within themselves.

NEGATIVE EMOTIONS: Defensive, aggressive, irritated, judgmental, making others wrong, egotistical, angry

POSITIVE PROPERTIES: Patient, rational, clear, secure, humble, willing to learn, considerate

COMPANION OILS: Citronella, Pink Pepper, Cardamom, Oregano, Tea Tree, Thyme, Amāvī®, Forgive

SUGGESTED USES:

Aromatic: Inhale from bottle, diffuse, or place drops in hand, rub, and inhale.

Topical: Dilute 1 drop with carrier oil and apply to the scalp or bottom of feet.

Environmental: Add several drops into spray bottle and mist around home.

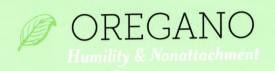

OREGANO
Humility & Nonattachment

Oregano cuts through the fluff of life and teaches individuals to do the same. It removes blocks, clears negativity, and cuts away negative attachments. Oregano is a powerful oil and may even be described as forceful or intense.

Oregano addresses the need to be right. Individuals in need of Oregano may attempt to convert other people to their own fixed opinions. Their strong will can make them unteachable and unwilling to budge. They hold rigidly to their opinions and belief systems. However, Oregano is resolute and has the power to break through a strong will and teach humility.

On the deepest level, Oregano dispels materialism and attachment that hinders growth and progress. While using Oregano, individuals may feel encouraged to end a toxic relationship, quit an oppressive job, or end a destructive habit. These toxic attachments limit the capacity to feel a healthy connection to the Divine. Oregano encourages true spirituality by inviting the soul to live in nonattachment and teaches that devotion to a Higher Power includes letting go of rigidity, willfulness, negative attachments, and materialism.

NEGATIVE EMOTIONS:
Negative attachments, prideful, opinionated, stubborn, materialistic, controlling

POSITIVE PROPERTIES: Humble, nonattachment, willing, teachable, flexible

COMPANION OILS: Sandalwood, Thyme, Tea Tree, Lemongrass, Cypress, Niaouli

SUGGESTED USES:
Aromatic: Inhale from bottle or diffuse and inhale.

Topical: Dilute 1 drop or less with carrier oil and apply on bottom of feet. **NOTE:** Use caution when applying topically.

Internal: Take 1-2 drops in a capsule, or in water.

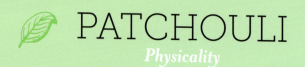

PATCHOULI
Physicality

Patchouli supports individuals in becoming fully present in their physical body. It balances those who feel devitalized and who seek to escape the body through spiritual pursuits or other forms of distraction. Patchouli tempers obsessive personalities by bringing them down to reality and teaching them moderation. This oil is grounding and stabilizing.

Patchouli complements yoga practice, tai chi, or other exercises that aim to connect the spirit with the body. While using Patchouli, individuals feel more grounded and fluid. This oil calms fear and nervous tension, stilling the heart and mind in preparing the spirit and body for deeper union. It also helps individuals to stay in touch with the earth.

Patchouli helps individuals appreciate the magnificence of the physical body and all of its natural processes and functions. It assists in releasing emotional judgments and issues related to the body, such as believing the body is unholy or dirty. This oil helps with body image distortions and general body dislike. Patchouli brings confidence in the body, as well as grace, poise, and physical strength. It reminds individuals of their childhood experiences when they used their bodies for play and fun. On the deepest level, Patchouli assists individuals to feel at peace while being present in their physical body.

NEGATIVE EMOTIONS:
Body shame and judgment, disconnected
from body, ungrounded, body tension

POSITIVE PROPERTIES:
Grounded, confident, moderation, body connection and acceptance, balanced, stable, physically expressive

COMPANION OILS: Grapefruit, Cinnamon

SUGGESTED USES:
Aromatic: Inhale from bottle, diffuse, or place drops in hand, rub, and inhale.
Topical: Apply 1-3 drops on bottom of feet or base of spine.
Internal: Take 1-2 drops under the tongue, in a capsule, or in water.

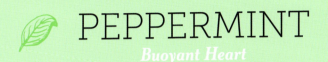

PEPPERMINT
Buoyant Heart

Peppermint brings joy and buoyancy to the heart and soul. It invigorates body, mind, and spirit, and reminds individuals that life can be happy, and they don't have to be controlled by fear. It lifts them out of their emotional trials for a short reprieve. When individuals use Peppermint, they feel as though they're gliding through life. It assists in staying on the surface of emotional issues like floating on top of water.

The power of Peppermint can be felt most in times of discouragement or despair. When individuals are disheartened, they may use Peppermint to rediscover the joy of being alive.

However, a person may also abuse the properties of Peppermint oil. If it is used as a permanent escape to avoid dealing with emotional pain, it can hinder growth and progress. Peppermint should not be used in this way. It aids individuals who need a short breather. At times, a reprieve is necessary before reentering emotional waters, but one is not meant to wade in the shallow end forever. When it is accepted and embraced, emotional pain serves as a teacher. Peppermint can assist individuals in regaining the strength needed to face their emotional reality.

NEGATIVE EMOTIONS: Unbearable anguish, intense despair, heavyhearted, pessimistic, sad

POSITIVE PROPERTIES: Buoyant, optimistic, relieved, strength to face emotional pain

COMPANION OILS: Tangerine, Elevation, Lime, Red Mandarin, Sunny Citrus, Island Mint®

SUGGESTED USES:
Aromatic: Inhale from bottle, diffuse, or place 1 drop in hand, rub, and inhale.

Topical: Dilute 1-2 drops with carrier oil and apply over chest, on shoulders, or back of neck.

Internal: Take 1-2 drops under the tongue, in a capsule, or in water.

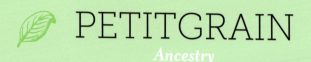

PETITGRAIN
Ancestry

Petitgrain invokes a deep appreciation for positive forms of ancestral knowledge, wisdom, and family history. All individuals carry a portion of their ancestors' lives and stories within them—physically, emotionally, and through inherited traditions. Petitgrain illuminates the eternal connection to all previous generations that weaves its way through the present generation and on to the next. It reminds individuals that it was by their ancestors' sacrifice they have the opportunity to experience this life. Petitgrain invites all to choose to honor the good that was inherited from their family and also make the path lighter for those who follow.

In this way, Petitgrain is also a great aid in healing a complicated family history. It invites individuals to accept the humanness of their ancestors and seek to learn from their mistakes. Instead of avoiding the pain of the past, Petitgrain encourages thoughtful awareness of how to heal wounds in the family line. It reveals patterns and tendencies of unconsciously repeating family mistakes. Individuals in need of Petitgrain may be unable or unwilling to depart from their family's way of thinking. Instead, they follow in the footsteps of their predecessors and ancestral traditions. Or they feel too bound to a family story they wish to disown and desire to disconnect from the reality of the previous generations. For either extreme, Petitgrain invites healthy awareness and balance. It encourages those who view any departure from tradition as a betrayal of the family to release the fear of disapproval and forge the path that is right for them. It also reminds those who desire to disconnect from their family origins to be willing to see the positives of healthy family connection. Petitgrain invites all to see the gift of their ancestral traditions and will assist them in their efforts to heal unfinished and unresolved ancestral issues.

Petitgrain reminds individuals that through accepting their ancestry, they can find peace, clarity, wisdom, and empathy for their own journey through this life.

NEGATIVE EMOTIONS: Disowning ancestry, repeating negative family patterns, duty-bound, loyal to unhealthy traditions, dishonoring progenitors

POSITIVE PROPERTIES: Pioneering, chain-breaking, cultivating healthy traditions, embracing positive family connections

COMPANION OILS: Siberian Fir, Birch, Douglas Fir, Bergamot

SUGGESTED USES:
Aromatic: Inhale from bottle or diffuse.

Topical: Dilute 1-3 drops with carrier oil and apply on bottom of feet or base of spine.

Internal: Take 1-2 drops under the tongue, in a capsule, or in water.

PINK PEPPER
Intrinsic Equality

Pink Pepper exposes the tendency of people to compare themselves to others. It challenges individuals to acknowledge their judgments of self and others generated by their comparisons. Oftentimes, individuals use judgment as a way to condemn the undesirable or disowned aspects of themselves. They don't recognize they are using external factors as a measuring stick of self-worth. Pink Pepper teaches that comparison never leads to happiness, but rather increases sorrow.

Most individuals are caught in a cycle of constant comparison by placing themselves either in a one-up or one-down position in every situation in their lives. The key to freedom is recognizing the tendency to overinflate the self at the expense of others, or conversely, of self-effacement at the expense of one's self. Pink Pepper energetically assists individuals with taking the middle path of equality found through their own self-acceptance.

Pink Pepper teaches that judgment and comparison are maladies of the heart. The only antidote to these insecurity-based behaviors is self-love and compassion. This oil catalyzes stagnant heart-space energies and moves the individual toward belief in the goodness of self, and ultimately, the belief in the goodness of others. Pink Pepper reminds that by being patient, kind, and loving to one's self, individuals can learn to extend that same mercy to those around them.

NEGATIVE EMOTIONS: Comparing, judgmental, unequal, distorted view of self

POSITIVE PROPERTIES: Equal, compassionate, accepting of self, kind, merciful

COMPANION OILS: Bergamot, Copaiba, Black Pepper, Geranium, Kumquat, Cassia, Forgive®, Niaouli

SUGGESTED USES:
Aromatic: Inhale from bottle or diffuse.
Topical: Dilute 1-2 drops with carrier oil and apply over chest and solar plexus (upper stomach).
Internal: Take 1-2 drops under the tongue, in a capsule, or in water.

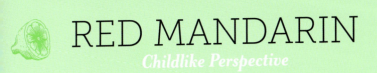

RED MANDARIN
Childlike Perspective

Mandarin is one of the parent fruits of all modern citrus varieties, and is considered to be one of the sweetest of all citrus fruits. As such, Red Mandarin oil offers a unique perspective: it invites individuals to see life through childlike eyes, appreciating the sweetness, wonder, and innocence in life. Children are not as easily set back or weighed down by the cares of life. They are quicker to move on and bounce back after encountering challenges. Red Mandarin invites adults to embrace this healthier, more resilient way of existing.

Red Mandarin can also be instrumental in supporting parenting. Oftentimes parents forget the magic and miracle of the lives they have created or accepted. The demands of day-to-day living, including the stress of providing for needs, addressing emotional upheavals, and sheer physical exhaustion can dim the joy, excitement, and purpose children can offer. Parents often find themselves feeling overwhelmed, unappreciated, and unable to meet the ever-present demands. This can lead to being discouraged, frustrated, angry, and filled with self-doubt. Red Mandarin reassures that while parenting can be extremely challenging, it can also be rewarding and refining.

This oil encourages all, parents and non-parents alike, to remember the innocence of childhood. It invites them to accept that the years of influence are short; life's seasons change, and children are constantly evolving, learning, and growing. Red Mandarin refreshes the weary and careworn parent and assists them to refocus on the beauty contained in the simple moments of life with a child. However, Red Mandarin reassures all who are overwhelmed that even though adult cares and concerns can be hard, life is still full of sweet moments that deserve to be noticed.

NEGATIVE EMOTIONS: Overwhelmed, weighed down, joyless parenthood, stressed, exhausted, discouraged, burdened, jaded

POSITIVE PROPERTIES: Seeing sweetness in life, wonder in parenting, refreshed, joy in simple moments, cherishing childhood, innocent, positive perspective

Myrrh, Frankincense, Serenity® ᵈᵒᵀᴱᴿᴿᴬ, Neroli, Ylang Ylang, Green Mandarin, Harvest Spice

SUGGESTED USES:

Aromatic: Inhale from bottle or diffuse.

Topical: Dilute 1-3 drops with carrier oil and apply around navel, on wrists, or behind ears.

Internal: Take 1-2 drops under the tongue, in a capsule, or in water.

YELLOW MANDARIN
From the unripe green mandarin to the mature red mandarin, this wonderful fruit provides plenty of emotional benefits in all its various stages. Yellow Mandarin occupies the middle stage, where individuals have already begun to evolve but have not yet seen their goals fulfilled. This oil helps in the literal and energetic in-between stages of life. It lifts the insecure and unsure. It also encourages individuals to think through their choices and look toward where they will eventually lead. Finally, Yellow Mandarin reminds all to inject plenty of friendliness and fun into the journey of becoming.

CLEMENTINE
The petite hybrid of orange and mandarin, Clementine represents sweetness in the small things. This oil reminds individuals not to miss the bliss of fleeting moments. Again and again, it is the littlest things in life that remind them they are blessed, loved, and cared for. Clementine teaches that everything one needs is often right before them, and to cherish the opportunity to savor the sweet simplicity of every moment.

ROMAN CHAMOMILE
Spiritual Purpose

Roman Chamomile supports individuals in discovering and living their true life's purpose. Regardless of what someone does for a living, they can find purpose and meaning in life. Purpose isn't defined simply by outward actions of individuals; it is housed within their heart and soul and radiates out to the world. As individuals live from the center of their beings, they find power and purpose that is indescribable. They also feel calmer and more at peace.

Roman Chamomile assists in shedding the meaningless activities that consume lives, so individuals can focus on a more fulfilling work, even the work of their own souls. This oil assists in feeling connected to and supported by divine helpers and guides, and calms insecurities about following one's spiritual path. When in doubt, Roman Chamomile softens the personality, easing the overactive ego-mind. It restores confidence in doing what they came to this earth to do. People fearfully believe that if they do what they love, they will end up destitute. Roman Chamomile reminds them to do what they love to experience true success.

NEGATIVE EMOTIONS: Purposeless, discouraged, drudgery, frustrated, unsettled

POSITIVE PROPERTIES: Purposeful, guided, peaceful, fulfilled, relaxed, spiritually connected

COMPANION OILS: Blue Tansy, Frankincense, Immortelle, Citrus Bloom

SUGGESTED USES:
Aromatic: Inhale from bottle, diffuse, or place drops in hand, rub, and inhale.

Topical: Apply 1-2 drops on forehead or behind ears.

Internal: Take 1-2 drops under the tongue, in a capsule, or in water.

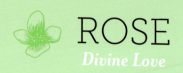

ROSE
Divine Love

Rose oil holds a higher vibration than any other oil on the planet. It is a powerful healer of the heart. It supports individuals in reaching heavenward and connecting with divine love. Rose teaches the essential need for divine grace and intervention in the healing process. As an individual opens to receive divine benevolence in all its manifestations, the heart is softened. If one can simply let go and choose to receive divine love, they are wrapped in warmth, charity, and compassion.

Rose invites individuals to experience the unwavering, unchanging, unconditional love of the Divine. This love heals all hearts and dresses all wounds. It restores individuals to authenticity, wholeness, and purity. As one feels unconditional love and acceptance, the heart is softened. As the heart fully opens, a fountain of love flows freely through the soul. In this state, one feels charity and compassion. Charity is experienced on behalf of oneself and others. Rose embodies divine love and teaches individuals how to contact this love through prayer, meditation, and opening the heart to receive.

NEGATIVE EMOTIONS: Bereft of divine love, constricted feelings, closed or broken heart, lack of compassion, wounded

POSITIVE PROPERTIES: Loved, compassionate, healing, tenderhearted, accepted, empathy, receiving divine love

COMPANION OILS: Geranium, Immortelle, Manuka, Arborvitae, Console®, Bergamot Mint

SUGGESTED USES:
Aromatic: Inhale from bottle or apply under nose.

Topical: Dilute 1 drop with carrier oil and apply over heart.

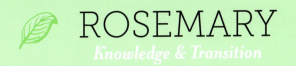

ROSEMARY
Knowledge & Transition

Rosemary assists in the development of true knowledge and true intellect. It teaches that one can be instructed from a far greater space of understanding than the human mind. It challenges individuals to look deeper than they normally would and ask more soul-searching questions so that they may receive more inspired answers.

Rosemary assists individuals who struggle with learning difficulties. It brings expansion to the mind, supporting individuals in receiving new information and new experiences.

Rosemary aids in times of transition and change. When a person is having a difficult time adjusting to a new house, school, or relationship, this oil can assist. Rosemary teaches that one does not understand all things with a mortal perspective.

It invites individuals to trust in a higher, more intelligent power than themselves. It supports them in feeling confident and assured during times of great change in understanding or perspective. Rosemary roots them in the true knowledge that surpasses all understanding.

NEGATIVE EMOTIONS: Confused, difficulty adjusting or transitioning, limited perspective, difficulties with learning

POSITIVE PROPERTIES: Mental clarity, knowledgeable, teachable, enlightened, open to new experiences, ability to adjust

COMPANION OILS: Dill, Lemon, Zendocrine®

SUGGESTED USES:
Aromatic: Inhale from bottle, diffuse, or place drops in hand, rub, and inhale.

Topical: Apply 1-3 drops on back of neck, forehead, or behind ears.

Internal: Take 1-2 drops under the tongue, in a capsule, or in water.

SANDALWOOD
Sacred Devotion

Sandalwood assists with all kinds of prayer, meditation, and spiritual worship. It teaches reverence and respect for Deity. This oil has been used since ancient times for its powerful ability to calm the mind, still the heart, and prepare the spirit to commune with God.

Sandalwood teaches of spiritual devotion and spiritual sacrifice. It invites individuals to place all material attachments on the altar of sacrifice so that they may truly progress spiritually. This oil asks them to assess where their hearts are and challenges them to reorder their priorities to be in alignment with the divine will.

Sandalwood assists in quieting the mind so that individuals may hear the subtle voice of the Spirit. It raises them into higher levels of consciousness. Sandalwood assists one in reaching beyond their current confines and belief systems. For those who are ready to leave behind attachment to fame, wealth, and the need for acceptance, Sandalwood teaches true humility, devotion, and love for the Divine.

NEGATIVE EMOTIONS:
Disconnected from God or spiritual self, emptiness, overthinking, materialistic

POSITIVE PROPERTIES: Humble, spiritual devotion, spiritual clarity, still, surrender, connected to higher consciousness

COMPANION OILS: Oregano, Spikenard, Immortelle, Peace®, Hinoki, Tulsi

SUGGESTED USES:
Aromatic: Inhale from bottle, diffuse, or place drops in hand, rub, and inhale before studying, meditating, or praying.

Topical: Apply 1 drop on crown of head or forehead.

Internal: Take 1-2 drops under the tongue, in a capsule, or in water.

NOTE: While there are several species of Sandalwood, both Hawaiian and Indian Sandalwood expand the sixth (brow) chakra. Hawaiian is slightly more supportive to additional upper chakra centers while Indian promotes slightly deeper and more ancient grounding in the lower chakras. They are both excellent oils for meditation and spiritual practices.

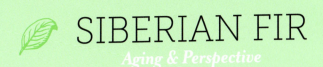

SIBERIAN FIR

Aging & Perspective

Siberian Fir addresses generational healing from the perspective of the mature. It assists during the twilight years as individuals transition into a more full, mature awareness. This period in one's life cycle can be beset with losses of many kinds. Siberian Fir offers comfort and support during periods of grief, regret, and longing. It aids in the necessary healing and reconciliation process of a life full of mixed experiences.

Siberian Fir encourages an honest and gentle approach to assessing one's life choices, influence, and legacy. Upon reflection, all people will find moments of regret and moments they cherish. Siberian Fir teaches that without the winds of opposition, individuals would never have gained the wisdom and strength they now possess. It also reminds that forgiveness—both needing to forgive and needing to be forgiven—is integral to development.

Siberian Fir helps ease difficult transitions by encouraging individuals to focus on finding meaning and purpose with each new chapter. As they progress through life, individuals may need to realign their hopes and aspirations to the realities of the present moment. Siberian Fir offers its steady energy through periods of change and adjustment, reminding individuals to look for the good and remember that they are inherently valuable and needed. The best gift that can be given to the next generation is sharing a heart at peace.

NEGATIVE EMOTIONS: Grieving, loss, despairing, sad, regretful, fretting over the past, pining

POSITIVE PROPERTIES: Comforted, forgiveness, perspective, honest, wisdom, living in the present, optimistic, adaptable, peaceful

COMPANION OILS: Arborvitae, Petitgrain, Forgive®, Peace®, Rosemary, Console®, Motivate®, Black Spruce

SUGGESTED USES:

Aromatic: Inhale from bottle, diffuse, or place drops in hand, rub, and inhale.

Topical: Apply 1-3 drops over heart, on wrists, or bottom of feet.

Internal: Take 1-2 drops under the tongue, in a capsule, or in water.

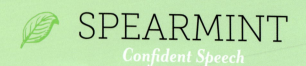

SPEARMINT
Confident Speech

Spearmint inspires clarity of thought and confident verbal expression. Individuals in need of Spearmint may hide their thoughts, opinions, and ideas by withholding their voices. Spearmint encourages inner clarity about one's personal convictions and opinions. It then assists individuals in translating that inner clarity into words.

Spearmint promotes confidence in expressing oneself verbally, especially when speaking in front of groups of people. It helps individuals create an effective stage presence by infusing them with confidence. Spearmint also encourages individuals to take a public stand on behalf of their values and opinions.

Spearmint can be a helpful remedy for those who struggle with communicating clearly for a wide range of reasons, from feeling scattered and inarticulate to stumbling over words. It assists individuals in becoming emotionally clear about what they want to say and then saying it. In short, Spearmint can help individuals access their inner light and convey that light to the world with clarity and confidence.

NEGATIVE EMOTIONS: Fear of public speaking, timid, holding back opinions, inarticulate

POSITIVE PROPERTIES: Confident, articulate communication, clarity, courageous

COMPANION OILS: Cassia, Lavender, Clary Sage, Laurel Leaf

SUGGESTED USES:
Aromatic: Inhale from bottle or diffuse.

Topical: Dilute 1-3 drops with carrier oil and apply over throat.

Internal: Take 1-2 drops under the tongue, in a capsule, or in water.

SPIKENARD
Gratitude

Spikenard encourages true appreciation for life. It addresses patterns of ingratitude, where individuals see themselves as targets of bad luck or victims of their life circumstances. This perception can often lead to feelings of blame and anger.

Spikenard encourages the soul to surrender and accept life exactly as it is. It invites individuals to let go and find an appreciation for all of life's experiences.

By opening the soul to acceptance and gratitude, Spikenard assists individuals in seeing the deeper meaning in their lives. It supports them in feeling joy and happiness for other people as well as for themselves. It invites individuals to expand by fully letting go of resistance, anger, and blame. Gratitude is an expression of complete acceptance and abundance. A grateful person is content with what they have. Spikenard teaches individuals to be grateful for their challenges as well as their blessings. It also assists individuals in transcending their sorrows through being grateful for their present life circumstances. Through complete surrender and acceptance, the soul may be brought into peace and harmony.

NEGATIVE EMOTIONS: Ungrateful, resisting, victim mentality, angry, greedy, selfish, expecting bad luck

POSITIVE PROPERTIES: Grateful, acceptance, content, peaceful

COMPANION OILS: Wild Orange, Immortelle, Lime, Ginger, Clove

SUGGESTED USES:
Aromatic: Inhale from bottle, diffuse, or place drops in hand, rub, and inhale.

Topical: Apply 1-3 drops on wrists, forehead, or over solar plexus (upper stomach).

STAR ANISE
Soulful Femininity

Star Anise has a warm, bolstering aroma that mirrors its emotional qualities. This plant embodies strong, calm, and reassuring energy. It enfolds all that one is, inviting all to come in to a sense of wholeness. From this state of wholeness, individuals are free to journey beyond where they have ever been before and learn to dance their heart song.

Star Anise is uplifting, balancing, and comforting to the careworn. It has the ability to be both flowing and consistent at the same time. It is helpful for reducing states of extreme contraction and moving individuals toward expansion. Star Anise guides the mind and body into a place of rest and regeneration before it reawakens them to rise and thrive again. If individuals are feeling worn down, this oil can reignite their inner spark, filling the fountain of their heart to overflowing once more. Star Anise reminds of the need for self-care, or for individuals to first stoke their inner fire, in order to send out unbridled love and strength to a world in need of what they bring.

Star Anise has a beautiful, feminine quality which works to strengthen and align female energy. Symbolically, Star Anise represents a sacred element and speaks to the soul energy on that plane. Its warm, nurturing embrace feels ancient and sacred. It reminds individuals that they are an empowered being of infinite worth.

NEGATIVE EMOTIONS: Incomplete, powerless, careworn, suppressed, weak, contracted, suppressed feminine power

POSITIVE PROPERTIES: Whole, powerful, reawakened, regenerated, thriving, calm, consistent, confident, expansive, strong, empowered femininity

COMPANION OILS: Cassia, Ginger, Whisper®, Myrrh, Cheer®, Rose, Davana

SUGGESTED USES:
Aromatic: Inhale from bottle or diffuse.
Topical: Dilute 1 drop or less with carrier oil and apply over solar plexus (upper stomach), sacral chakra (lower stomach), and heart. **NOTE:** Use caution when applying topically.
Internal: Take 1-2 drops under the tongue, in a capsule, or in water.

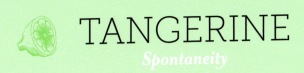

TANGERINE
Spontaneity

Tangerine's strong qualities of joyfulness can lift the darkest of moods. It can assist those who feel cut off from the lightness of heart often manifested by children. Those who feel overburdened by responsibility would benefit from Tangerine's uplifting vibration. It encourages a person to be creative and spontaneous.

Creativity can be stifled by an excessive sense of duty or creating rigid standards for oneself. While work, duty, and responsibility all have their place, feeling overworked, overly responsible, and overburdened leads to a loss of creative energy. Tangerine invites individuals to make room for their creative side, and asks that they reinsert fun, joy, and spontaneity into their lives.

Tangerine supports individuals in accessing the abundant pool of creative energy held within the spirit. It then assists that energy in flowing through the heart and into physical manifestation. Tangerine teaches individuals to enjoy life by being more abundantly creative and to re-experience the joy and spontaneity they knew in childhood.

NEGATIVE EMOTIONS: Overburdened by responsibilities, stifled creativity, duty-bound, overworked, heavyhearted, joyless

POSITIVE PROPERTIES: Creative, spontaneous, fun, fulfilled, lighthearted, joyful, happy, optimistic

COMPANION OILS: Cheer®, Citrus Bliss®, Ylang Ylang, Basil, Wild Orange, Lime, Sunny Citrus, Red Mandarin, Green Mandarin, Harvest Spice, Davana

SUGGESTED USES:
Aromatic: Inhale from bottle, diffuse, or place drops in hand, rub, and inhale.

Topical: Apply 1-2 drops on wrists, over heart, or sacral chakra (lower stomach).

Internal: Take 1-2 drops under the tongue, in a capsule, or in water.

TEA TREE
Energetic Boundaries

A cleanser by nature, Tea Tree, also known as tea tree oil, clears negative energetic baggage. It specifically releases codependent and parasitic relationships. These toxic relationships may be with people, microorganisms in the physical body, or spiritual beings. Individuals may feel drained of life force and energy, but they may not be consciously aware of the source of this energy leakage. Tea Tree helps break the negative ties in these kinds of relationships so that new, healthy connections may be formed that honor one's personal space and boundaries. This energetic "vampirism" between organisms violates the laws of nature. Tea Tree encourages an individual to connect to people and beings in ways that honor and respect others' agency. It helps individuals recognize the parts of themselves that invited and allowed these kinds of relationships to exist in the first place.

Through these empowering processes, Tea Tree encourages individuals to relinquish all forms of self-betrayal, including allowing others to take advantage of one's time, energy, or talents; letting others feed on one's energy; not standing up for oneself; or feeling responsible for the problems of others. Tea Tree assists individuals in purification practices and in releasing toxic debris.

NEGATIVE EMOTIONS: Parasitic and codependent relationships, poor boundaries, weak-willed, drained, emotional toxicity, powerless

POSITIVE PROPERTIES: Energetic boundaries, healthy and respectful connections, empowered, resilient, safe

COMPANION OILS: Clove, TerraShield®, On Guard®, Lemongrass, Lemon Myrtle, Yarrow | Pom, Niaouli

SUGGESTED USES:
Aromatic: Inhale from bottle, diffuse, or place drops in hand, rub, and inhale.

Topical: Apply 1-3 drops on bottom of feet or the crown of the head.

Environmental: Add several drops into spray bottle and mist around home.

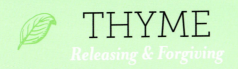

THYME
Releasing & Forgiving

Thyme is one of the most powerful cleansers of the emotional body and assists in addressing trapped feelings which have been buried for a long time. It reaches deep within the body and soul, searching for unresolved negativity. Thyme brings to the surface old, stagnant feelings. It is particularly helpful in treating the toxic emotions of hate, rage, anger, and resentment, which cause the heart to close.

Thyme empties the soul of negativity, leaving the heart wide open. In this state of openness, individuals begin to feel tolerance and patience for others. As the heart opens more and more, it is able to receive love and offer forgiveness. Thyme teaches that it's time to let go and move forward. As individuals forgive, they free themselves from emotional bondage. Thyme transforms hate and anger into love and forgiveness.

NEGATIVE EMOTIONS: Unforgiving, angry, raging, hateful, bitter, resentful, emotional bondage

POSITIVE PROPERTIES: Forgiving, tolerant, patient, openhearted, understanding, emotional release

COMPANION OILS: Cardamom, Forgive®, Geranium, Cypress, Oregano, Niaouli

SUGGESTED USES:
Aromatic: Inhale from bottle or diffuse.

Topical: Dilute 1 drop or less with carrier oil and apply on chest, over sacral chakra (lower stomach), or on bottom of feet. **NOTE**: Use caution when applying topically.

Internal: Take 1-2 drops under the tongue, in a capsule, or in water.

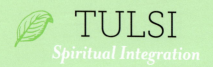

TULSI
Spiritual Integration

Tulsi, or Holy Basil, is a sacred and highly valued herb in India. It is considered indispensable, as nothing compares with its majestic qualities. It has a host of beneficial uses including being a powerful adaptogen for many body systems, acting to balance and restore areas that have become weakened or blocked. It enhances prana—or life force energy—and restores energetic flow for healing body, mind, and spirit.

Tulsi aids in harmonizing the conscious and unconscious mind. This unified energy meets in the center, or heart, of one's being. This exceptionally high vibration oil shifts negative mental and emotional states almost instantly. It is excellent for individuals feeling overcome by stress and emotional dysregulation. It penetrates the deepest emotional wounds and offers an invitation to heal what remains unresolved or previously unreachable. This oil is a powerful ally for healing the heart and choosing into one's emotional work.

Tulsi's greatest influence is on the spiritual and energetic plane. It reveals the often unseen strain of living out of alignment with one's spiritual purpose. It reminds individuals—on a soul-level—of their purpose which existed before they manifested physically on this earth. It helps them release their resistance to life and spiritually integrate for full actualization. Tulsi is an indispensable aid in spiritual awakening.

NEGATIVE EMOTIONS: Misaligned, weakened, energetically blocked, strained, stressed

POSITIVE PROPERTIES: Integrated, alive, energetically clear, harmonized, balanced, healed

COMPANION OILS: Sandalwood, Clary Sage, Basil, Immortelle, DDR Prime, Copaiba, Magnolia, Melissa

SUGGESTED USES:

Aromatic: Inhale from bottle, diffuse, or place drops in hand, rub, and inhale.

Topical: Dilute 1 drop with carrier oil and apply on crown of head and temples.

TURMERIC

Restoration

Turmeric repairs individuals physically, mentally, and emotionally. It has powerful properties that reach into damaged or blocked aspects of the self to restore what has been temporarily lost. Turmeric is a powerful antidote for those who feel paralyzed by the inherent dangers of life, or by a loss of function or freedom they once took for granted. It is particularly beneficial when one feels weighed down due to personal tragedies or loss of confidence in abilities. Turmeric offers strength and hope to ground individuals during times of upheaval or significant change.

Turmeric can also restore one's faith in goodness. It reminds that for good or bad, each person occupies a unique role in the unfolding destiny of the world. In a season where atrocities are committed and heartless events unfold without meaning or seeming consequence, exposure to the misdeeds of others can cause faith in humankind to grow cold. Turmeric restores belief that most individuals choose to act as agents for good—despite the associated risks. The strong warmth of turmeric provides stability for the wavering heart and a foundation of trust that people are capable of good and progress is always possible.

Turmeric also assists those who struggle against systemic barriers such as prejudice, bias, and racism by helping individuals recognize discordant or damaging messages and distinguish them from the truth. Turmeric imbues the soul with courage and lends the strength to turn what seem like unconquerable obstacles into navigable paths.

NEGATIVE EMOTIONS: Damaged, unsteady, abused, oppressed, afraid, betrayed, hopeless, paralyzed

POSITIVE PROPERTIES: Faithful, resilient, confident, grounded, stable, restored, believing, trusting

COMPANION OILS: Ginger, Litsea, Fennel, Cassia, Blue Tansy, Hope®, Laurel Leaf

SUGGESTED USES:

Aromatic: Inhale from bottle, diffuse, or place drops in hand, rub, and inhale.

Topical: Apply 1-2 drops on forehead, over solar plexus (upper stomach), or on bottom of feet.

Internal: Take 1-2 drops under the tongue, in a capsule, or in water.

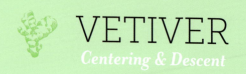

VETIVER
Centering & Descent

Vetiver oil assists in becoming more rooted in life. Life can scatter one's energy and make individuals feel split between different priorities, people, and activities. Vetiver brings the individual back down to earth. It assists in grounding to the physical world. Vetiver also assists individuals in deeply connecting with what they think and feel. In this way, Vetiver is incredibly supportive in all kinds of self-awareness work. It helps uncover the root of an emotional issue.

Vetiver challenges the need to escape pain. It centers individuals in their True Self and guides them downward to the root of their emotional issues. It helps them find relief but not through avoidance. Relief comes after they have traveled within and met the core of their emotional issue. Vetiver will not let them quit. It grounds them in the present moment and carries them through an emotional catharsis. The descent into the True Self assists individuals in discovering deeper facets of their being. Vetiver opens the doors to light and recovery through this downward journey.

NEGATIVE EMOTIONS: Apathetic, disconnected, scattered, stressed, ungrounded, avoiding, crisis

POSITIVE PROPERTIES: Centered, grounded, present, emotionally aware and connected

COMPANION OILS: Helichrysum, Juniper Berry, Balance®, Hinoki

SUGGESTED USES:
Aromatic: Inhale from bottle, diffuse, or place drops in hand, rub, and inhale.

Topical: Apply 1-3 drops on bottom of feet or base of spine.

Internal: Take 1-2 drops under the tongue, in a capsule, or in water.

WILD ORANGE
Abundance

Wild Orange addresses a wide variety of emotional issues. It inspires abundance, fosters creativity, and supports a positive mood. Wild Orange also reconnects individuals with their inner child and brings spontaneity, fun, joy, and playfulness into one's life.

At its core, Wild Orange teaches the true meaning of abundance. It encourages individuals to let go of a scarcity mindset with all of its manifestations, including fear, nervousness, inflexibility, workaholism, lack of humor, and the belief that there is not enough. Wild Orange reminds the soul of the limitless supply found in nature. Fruit trees, like the orange tree, give freely to all in need. This oil teaches individuals to give without thought of compensation. In nature, there is always enough to go around. Wild Orange encourages individuals to let go of their need to hoard, which is the epitome of scarcity.

Wild Orange also assists an individual's natural creative sense. It inspires limitless solutions for problems and issues. One never needs to live in fear. Wild Orange invites individuals to completely let go as a child does and to live from their True Self. At a person's core, there is abundance. Sharing, playing, relaxing, and enjoying the bounties of life—these are the gifts bestowed by Wild Orange oil.

NEGATIVE EMOTIONS: Scarcity, overly serious, rigid, dull, workaholic, lack of energy, discouraged, hoarding, envious

POSITIVE PROPERTIES: Abundant, sense of humor, playful, generous, spontaneous, creative, joyful

COMPANION OILS: Tangerine, Lemon, Ylang Ylang, Red Mandarin, Citrus Bloom®, Davana

SUGGESTED USES:
Aromatic: Inhale from bottle, diffuse, or place drops in hand, rub, and inhale.

Topical: Apply 1-3 drops over sacral chakra (lower stomach).

Internal: Take 1-2 drops under the tongue, in a capsule, or in water.

WINTERGREEN
Surrender

Wintergreen is the oil of surrender. It can assist strong-willed individuals in letting go of the need to know and the need to be right. It takes great internal strength to surrender to a Higher Power. Wintergreen imbues the soul with this strength and teaches how to let go and be free of the negativity and pain one holds on to. The belief that life is painful and must be shouldered alone makes it so. Wintergreen invites individuals to surrender these strong opinions.

Wintergreen reminds individuals that they do not have to do life on their own. There is a constant invitation to surrender one's burdens to a Higher Power. All that is required is to release and let go. Wintergreen teaches that one can turn their hardships over to that power greater than themselves so they do not have to carry the burden of life all alone.

NEGATIVE EMOTIONS: Controlling, willful, needing to be right, burdened, excessive self-reliance

POSITIVE PROPERTIES: Surrender, relying on divine grace, nonattachment, teachable, strengthened

COMPANION OILS: Sandalwood, Oregano, Frankincense, Arborvitae

SUGGESTED USES:
Aromatic: Inhale from bottle or diffuse.

Topical: Dilute 1-2 drops with carrier oil and apply over heart.

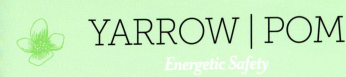

YARROW | POM
Energetic Safety

Yarrow is a conduit for light and creates feelings of emotional and energetic safety. It serves as an oil of protection by shielding individuals from negative influences that drain energy and strength. These influences may be from other individuals or world events, as well as unseen spiritual forces that may be at play in their lives. In this way, Yarrow has the ability to dispel feelings of darkness that can overshadow individuals with anxiousness, worry, and fear.

Yarrow can also help harmonize one's energy system following crisis or trauma. Its regenerative properties assist in balancing chemistry, purifying stagnant chi, and increasing receptivity to positive influences. Regardless of the negative energy or incident, Yarrow can help an individual feel more protected, strengthened, and rejuvenated.

Yarrow is also extremely helpful in discerning light from dark. It encourages opening to love and connection when an individual has become too closed, protected, or fearful. Yarrow reassures that the Divine is near, is upholding all things, and desires the safety and protection for all on their journey through life.

Combining Yarrow with Pomegranate adds a layer of depth and complexity that amplifies the emotional properties. Pomegranate has long been revered as a sacred plant by many cultures, symbolizing humanity's central beliefs and ideals about life, death, learning, wisdom, and fruitfulness. Pomegranate brings in an added spiritual element that marries with Yarrow beautifully.

NEGATIVE EMOTIONS: Unsafe, unclear, unprotected, fearful, energetically weakened, attacked, weak boundaries, in crisis, overwhelmed, scattered

POSITIVE PROPERTIES: Protected, discerning, strong boundaries, safe, assisted, open, centered, clear, ability to relax and receive, balance, peace

COMPANION OILS: Tea Tree, Frankincense, On Guard®, TerraShield®, Melissa

SUGGESTED USES:

Aromatic: Inhale from bottle, diffuse, or place drops in hand, rub, and inhale.

Topical: Apply 1 drop on crown of head or base of spine.

Environmental: Add several drops into a spray bottle and mist around home.

Internal: Take 1-2 drops under the tongue, in a capsule, or in water.

YLANG YLANG
Inner Child

Ylang Ylang is a powerful remedy for the heart. Modern-day society honors and reveres the mind over the heart. Yet the heart, with its intuitive ways of receiving information, is an essential part of the soul. Ylang Ylang reconnects individuals with the inner child and the pure, simple ways of the heart. It encourages play and restores a childlike nature and innocence. It assists in accessing intuition or heart-knowing.

Ylang Ylang is also a powerful remedy for releasing emotional trauma from the past. It is a fantastic support in age regression work and other methods of emotional healing. Ylang Ylang also assists individuals in releasing bottled-up emotions such as anger and sadness. Feelings that have been buried inside are brought to the light through Ylang Ylang's assistance. This oil allows emotional healing to flow naturally, nurturing the heart through the process. It reminds the individual that joy can be felt and experienced more fully by allowing the heart its full range of emotions.

NEGATIVE EMOTIONS: Joyless, stressed, overanalyzing, sad, disconnected from inner child

POSITIVE PROPERTIES: Playful, free, intuitive, emotionally connected, healing, joyful, innocent

COMPANION OILS: Geranium, Tangerine, Wild Orange, Rose, Red Mandarin, Bergamot Mint

SUGGESTED USES:
Aromatic: Inhale from bottle, diffuse, or place drops in hand, rub, and inhale.

Topical: Apply 1-3 drops over heart.

Internal: Take 1-2 drops under the tongue, in a capsule, or in water.

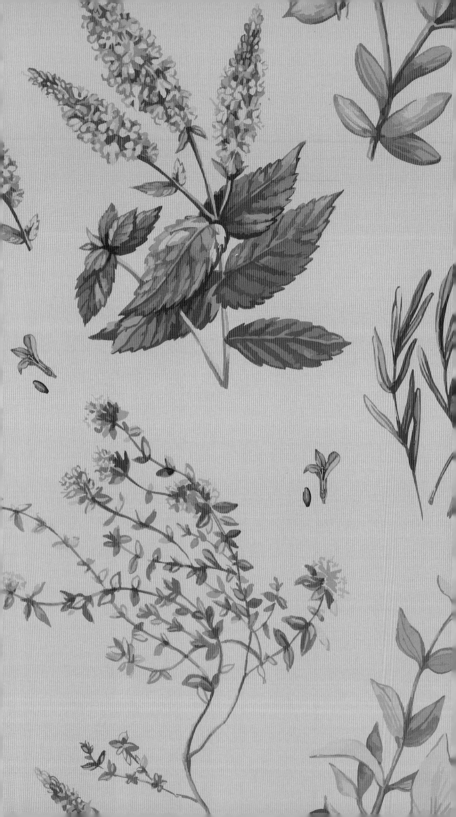

OIL BLENDS

Oil blends are created by combining several single oils to form an entirely new synergy greater than the sum of its parts. Blends are formulated to address specific physical or emotional themes or issues, and can assist with your healing by increasing the variety of emotional states addressed. Oil blends are unique from single oils but not necessarily superior. Still, blends may be more equipped than single oils because of their dynamic nature. Oil blends multiply effectiveness to address targeted issues.

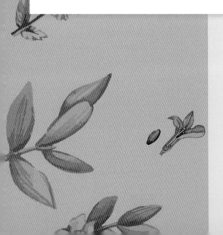

ADAPTIV®
Adaptability

Adaptiv® was formulated to assist with anxious states. It imparts reassurance and calm when one is caught in cycles of constriction, tension, worry, solicitude, or uneasiness. When individuals have experienced prolonged stress or traumatic experiences, the mind-body responds by becoming hypervigilant in order to protect them from future harm. This state is antithetical to well-being and positive functioning. Adaptiv® helps individuals adapt to stressors and fears in more clear, constructive, and confident ways.

Adaptiv® invites individuals to look deeper into the messages behind their emotional manifestations and examine where these reactions may be stemming from. It teaches them to recognize the parts of themselves that need to be given a voice. This blend will partner with individuals in asking the difficult questions of why they don't feel safe and what part of themselves is in need of attention. It cautions that self-judgment and self-loathing are functions of the inner critic and only inflict further trauma on an already overwhelmed soul. Adaptiv® teaches the need for kindness toward one's self and self-acceptance for wherever they are on their journey.

Adaptiv® conveys softly the truth that most of life is beyond the ability to control, and safety is only to be found in the arms of the Divine. It reminds the weary soul that the Divine has always and will always be there, holding, caring for, and loving them. The invitation from this blend is to not take another step alone when divine love is offering its grace, compassion, and refuge to lean in to. Adaptiv® asks individuals to exercise faith that they will be carried when they no longer know the way and to believe they are never alone.

INGREDIENTS: Wild Orange, Lavender, Copaiba, Spearmint, Neroli, Sweetgum, Laurel Leaf

NEGATIVE EMOTIONS: Anxious, uneasy, worried, self-critical, obsessing, controlling, fearful

POSITIVE PROPERTIES: Reassured, calm, clear, confident, self-acceptance, liberated, trusting, upheld, safe

SUGGESTED USES:
Aromatic: Inhale from bottle, diffuse, or place drops in hand, rub, and inhale.

Topical: Apply over chest, stomach, or on forehead.

ALIGN
Centering

Align calls the soul back to its center. It reaches gently into the heart space to shift heavy energies that are inhibiting progress and disrupting stillness and flow. While working on the heart center, it recalibrates an individual's inherent integrity and brings into awareness the costs of misalignment. It reminds that self-awareness, even if temporarily unpleasant, is the gateway to further expansion and growth. This blend invites individuals to pause and practice self-acceptance during moments of self-reflection, which allows them to act from a more conscious and clear space.

Align facilitates the emergence of love, openness, and trust. It encourages individuals to live congruently and offer true generosity to others. This blend invites individuals to refrain from projecting onto others' inaccurate or unkind motives and instead allows for a reflection of goodness to manifest in those with whom they come in contact. It can be difficult to choose this higher path when one has been repeatedly let down by the choices of others. However, this blend teaches that fearlessly choosing to stay open is the only way to stay in alignment. Align restores emotional balance by reorienting the heart back to its state of true purpose: love.

INGREDIENTS: Bergamot, Coriander, Marjoram, Peppermint, Geranium, Basil, Rose, Jasmine

NEGATIVE EMOTIONS: Misaligned, confused, conflicted, out of integrity, imbalanced, closed, distrusting, divided energies, fractured

POSITIVE PROPERTIES: Centered, aligned, still, integrity, self-acceptance, open-minded, trusting, loving

SUGGESTED USES:
Aromatic: Inhale from bottle, diffuse, or place drops in hand, rub, and inhale.

Topical: Apply to chest, stomach, or middle chakras (mid-back).

AMĀVĪ®
Balanced Masculine

Amāvī® offers protective, meditative, and deeply grounding energy. This stability supports individuals to gather the necessary strength to face challenges and remain calm in adversity. This blend reminds that true strength lies not in outward facades, or expressions of egotism or dominance, but rather in connecting to one's own inner guidance and acting out of integrity.

Amāvī® encourages softening, purifying, and opening of the heart to assist in experiencing emotional clarity and honesty. It persuades individuals to release demanding expectations and false paradigms which drive them to perfectionism, control, anxiousness, irritability, workaholism, escapism, and stress. This blend invites all to slow down, breathe, relax, reconnect to their bodies, and simply be.

Amāvī® is also excellent for addressing male generational patterns and strained relationships with men. If individuals have rejected the masculine, isolated from men, or conversely, become overly masculine, this blend invites them to connect with healthy masculine energy, which is calm, grounded, aware, and strong, and to return to balance. Amāvī® assists both men and women in aligning with balanced male energy.

INGREDIENTS: Buddha Wood, Balsam Fir Wood, Black Pepper, Hinoki, Patchouli, Cocoa Extract, Niaouli

NEGATIVE EMOTIONS: Challenged, dominant, egotistical, stressed, resistant to male energy, resistant to men

POSITIVE PROPERTIES: Stable, strong, strengthened, calm, integrity, accepting of the masculine, balanced male energy, emotional clarity

SUGGESTED USES:
Aromatic: Inhale from bottle, diffuse, or place drops in hand, rub, and inhale.

Topical: Apply on bottom of feet, over chest, on back of neck, and along spine.

ANCHOR
Steadying

Anchor offers steadiness to individuals when they experience upheaval or instability, either in their outward or inward life. Its calm, present, and supportive aroma extends an energetic arm to lean on. When an individual is being invited by life to accept radical change, it is common to look externally for support and reassurance when faith in oneself falters. However, Anchor invites individuals to look inward to discover the refuge that is already within reach. It is supportive for individuals who wish to practice trusting their intuition and accepting the wisdom waiting within their own soul.

Anchor reminds that separateness, uncertainty, and concealment are symptoms of fear and not solutions. This blend invites individuals to remain present and aware when they feel the pull to choose out of integrity and self-protect. It teaches them to return to trust and find their center one moment at a time. Anchor encourages individuals to step onto the path before them with faith and courage, offering reassurance that it will be there, holding space, for as long as it's needed.

INGREDIENTS: Lavender, Cedarwood, Frankincense, Cinnamon, Sandalwood, Black Pepper, Patchouli

NEGATIVE EMOTIONS: Unsteady, upheaval, uncertain, separated

POSITIVE PROPERTIES: Steady, calm, present, supported, clear, courageous

SUGGESTED USES:
Aromatic: Inhale from bottle, diffuse, or place drops in hand, rub, and inhale.

Topical: Apply over chest, stomach, or middle chakras (mid-back).

ARISE
Enlightening

Arise invites individuals to rise up and meet their life. This blend teaches that most individuals are living well beneath their potential. It invites them to choose—in this moment—to reclaim the fullness they were always meant to experience. This blend expands the soul and helps it to realize it is capable of more than it ever thought possible.

Arise can powerfully lift despondent or burdened individuals and fill them with enthusiasm, joy, and optimism. It raises the vibration of an individual into states of light, creation, and manifestation, which allows stagnant energy to dissolve naturally.

Arise reawakens intuition and insight. It encourages the full acceptance of all parts of the soul—mind, body, and spirit—so that in wholeness and unity they may ascend together. Arise catalyzes the sparks of divinity within everyone that long to reconnect to the Divine and arise to their full potential.

INGREDIENTS: Lemon, Grapefruit, Siberian Fir, Osmanthus, and Melissa

NEGATIVE EMOTIONS: Burdened, joyless, pessimistic, fragmented, spiritually disconnected

POSITIVE PROPERTIES: Integrated, intuitive, lifted, joyful, enthusiastic, optimistic, actualized

SUGGESTED USES:
Aromatic: Inhale from bottle, diffuse, or place drops in hand, rub, and inhale.

Topical: Apply on forehead, crown of head, or upper chakras (back of neck).

AROMATOUCH®
Relaxation

AromaTouch® assists the body in calming, relaxing, and releasing physical tension. On an emotional level, AromaTouch® moves an individual from stiffness of heart and mind to openness and flexibility. This blend is soothing to both body and mind, and offers comfort in times of grief and sorrow.

Most people seek out massage when they are tense or stressed. Through bodywork and massage, individuals are able to relax tight muscles. Breathing may begin to regulate, slow, and deepen. As the body relaxes, so does the mind. As muscles release tension, the heart can reopen to life. Circulation is enhanced, as is one's ability to move with life and allow things to flow. This is the gift of AromaTouch®— the ability to relax, open, and move in harmony once more with the body and with existence.

INGREDIENTS: Cypress, Peppermint, Marjoram, Basil, Grapefruit, Lavender

NEGATIVE EMOTIONS: Tense, stressed, rigid, unable to relax, inflexible

POSITIVE PROPERTIES: Relaxed, balanced, flexible, comforted, open mind and heart

SUGGESTED USES:
Aromatic: Inhale from bottle, diffuse, or place drops in hand, rub, and inhale.

Topical: Massage 1-3 drops wherever emotional or physical tension is experienced.

BALANCE®
Grounding

Balance® is primarily a combination of tree oils and roots. Trees live in the present moment. They are not in a hurry; they are stable. The soft energy of Balance® is excellent for calming overactive children who have difficulty settling down. It is also a wonderful remedy for those who need to reconnect with their roots. Balance® strengthens a connection with the lower body and with the earth. These connections are especially important when the upper faculties have been overused due to excessive thinking, speaking, or spiritual activity.

Balance® is especially suited for personalities who seek to escape from life through disconnection or disassociation. These individuals may avoid long-term commitments in work or relationships, preferring instead to drift. This blend reminds individuals that to realize their true dreams and desires, they must stay focused on a goal until it is actualized in the physical world. Balance® teaches true perseverance by assisting in staying present with a specific plan or idea until it is embodied. Providing inner strength and fortitude, Balance® teaches all to ground their energy and to manifest their vision with the patience of a tree.

INGREDIENTS: Spruce, Ho Wood, Frankincense, Blue Tansy, Blue Chamomile, Osmanthus

NEGATIVE EMOTIONS: Scattered, ungrounded, disconnected, unstable

POSITIVE PROPERTIES: Grounded, stable, connected, committed, self-contained, inner strength, persevering

SUGGESTED USES:
Aromatic: Inhale from bottle, diffuse, or place drops in hand, rub, and inhale.

Topical: Apply 1-3 drops on base of spine or bottom of feet.

BEAUTIFUL
Self-Respect

Beautiful was formulated to uplift the mood and encourage self-confidence and self-respect. This combination of oils beautifully unfolds the heart space, reopening it to love and self-acceptance.

Too often inherent value is gauged from outward responses instead of inner knowing. The oils in Beautiful lead individuals to recognize the beauty of the gifts within them and to embrace their worth with grace and gratitude. It can be easier to find personal faults than to find inner strengths, talents, and capabilities. This blend helps individuals acknowledge all that is good within and to radiate their divine light to a world in need.

Beautiful can also provide clarity about the things that captivate individuals. It encourages an honest assessment of where an individual places value and what influences are allowed into one's life. It gently lifts the eyes to meet the truth about present circumstances. It helps develop an innate sense of what is good and trustworthy, and when priorities are out of alignment, them the strength to let go of relationships, beliefs, and behaviors that aren't serving the highest good.

Beautiful is a soothing heart tonic for those whose beauty has been used as an instrument against them. If individuals have been taken advantage of, abused, or misused, this blend wraps them in layer upon layer of love and sanctuary. It reminds them that they are worthy and fully loved; they are safe to be seen and their beauty has never been, and can never be, diminished by outside forces. It promises that when sorrows have been grieved, love will return as a healer.

INGREDIENTS: Lime, Osmanthus, Bergamot and, Frankincense

NEGATIVE EMOTIONS: Abused, self-loathing, self-critical, misused, unworthy, grieving

POSITIVE PROPERTIES: Self-confident, self-love, self-respect, graceful, grateful, beautiful, capable, lovable, soothed, healing, worthy

SUGGESTED USES:
Aromatic: Inhale from bottle or diffuse.

Topical: Apply over heart, center of chest, on neck, or behind ears.

BRAVE®
Courage

Brave® invites individuals to treat others with mutual respect, which includes respect for the self. There is an opportunity in every communication to choose to honor the humanity of each person, as every soul is deserving of nothing less. It helps those who have struggled with being mistreated, bullied, excluded, or made to feel less than others. This blend also imbues them with the tenacity to confront the untruths they have believed about themselves because of negative experiences. Brave® clears emotional debris, bolstering individuals with the knowledge that their worth can never be devalued by the actions of others.

Brave® encourages all to speak up or speak out against things that are wrong, either with their peers or in their family, especially if they feel the problem is theirs to shoulder alone. It takes courage to be vulnerable and share what one has been afraid to say. However, it is through this intrepidity they will free themselves from the destructive consequences of concealment. Brave® blend confronts the lie that keeping something hidden keeps it safe. It is only through standing up for the truth, no matter how frightening it may seem, that the individual can step firmly back into the light and be free. Brave® Blend invites all to reclaim the courage they lack. It teaches the only power fear has is the power it is given.

INGREDIENTS: Wild Orange, Amyris, Osmanthus, Cinnamon

NEGATIVE EMOTIONS: Afraid, less than, bullied, hiding, unsure

POSITIVE PROPERTIES: Courageous, respectful, worthy, resolute

SUGGESTED USES:

Aromatic: Inhale from bottle, diffuse, or place drops in hand, rub, and inhale.

Topical: Apply 1-3 drops over solar plexus (upper stomach)..

NOTE: As children learn to find their courage through life's everyday moments, Brave® is an excellent companion, whether reciting something from memory, facing a challenging situation, or stepping into a ballgame.

BREATHE®

Breath

Breathe® addresses the inability to let go of grief and pain. Individuals in need of Breathe® struggle to take breath and literally feel suffocated by sadness. The lungs and air passages become constricted, preventing air and emotion from releasing. The root of this condition is feeling unloved; individuals grieve the love they never received. They often shut down due to fear, not knowing whether the love they need will be there. They distrust whether it's safe to open and take in life. Breathe® encourages individuals to release grief and sadness and to receive genuine love and healing.

Breathe® also supports one's relationship with spirit and deepens one's connection to life. It invites individuals to let go (breathe out) and receive (breathe in). In this way, this blend teaches individuals to embrace life through breath. Breathe® imbues individuals with the courage to fully open.

INGREDIENTS: Laurel (Bay), Eucalyptus, Peppermint, Tea Tree, Lemon, Cardamom, Ravensara

NEGATIVE EMOTIONS: Sad, grieving, despairing, unloved, constricted, distrusting, closed

POSITIVE PROPERTIES: Loved, supported, receiving, open, healing, solace, embracing life, trusting

SUGGESTED USES:
Aromatic: Inhale from bottle or diffuse, or place drops in hand, rub and inhale.

Topical: Dilute 1-3 drops with carrier oil and apply over heart or chest.

CALMER®
Restful

Calmer® has a soothing influence on the heart and mind. It consoles individuals when they are feeling out of control, worried, or overwhelmed. This blend is also beneficial when an individual is feeling overstimulated and has trouble quieting the mind and restoring inner harmony. Trying to do too much in life or fit too much in each day is disquieting to the delicate inner workings of most individuals. Calmer® is stabilizing and reassuring when the frenetic pace of life disturbs one's center.

Calmer® blend gently encourages individuals to look for patterns of imbalance that may be playing out in their lives and to choose to realign with their intuition and heart-knowing. It reminds that while there are many good things that one can choose to spend their time on, there are actually very few that will bring lasting happiness, peace, and purpose. They can choose each new day to slow down and check within to discover what it is that they should embrace and what they should let go of.

On its deepest level, Calmer® invites individuals to trust in the divine will trying to manifest in their lives. It helps in feeling connected to and supported by divine beings of light. Calmer® speaks softly its comforting, core message: everything is going to be okay.

INGREDIENTS: Lavender, Cananga (Ylang Ylang flower), Buddha Wood, Roman Chamomile

NEGATIVE EMOTIONS: Upset, worried, over-scheduled, imbalanced, frenetic

POSITIVE PROPERTIES: Calm, reassured, restful, realigned, peaceful

SUGGESTED USES:
Aromatic: Inhale from bottle, diffuse, or place drops in hand, rub, and inhale.

Topical: Apply 1-3 drops over heart, on forehead, or back of neck.

NOTE: To help a child wind down at bedtime or ease their emotions and temperament, or to soothe a fussy baby, Calmer(R) oil blend supports little ones of all ages.

> NOTE: The Kids Collection was specifically formulated with smaller bodies in mind, with each blend purposely diluted to offer a softer, more gentle experience. These formulations also work well for those with fragile health or skin, or who are highly sensitive. They serve both young and old alike.

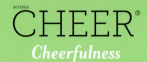

CHEER®
Cheerfulness

This blend of citruses and spices was formulated to assist those who are in need of cheerfulness. It is especially helpful for individuals who feel heavyhearted or who have been weighed down by many challenges in life. Encountering repeated trials over an extended period of time can have crippling effects, and may even create an expectation of permanent suffering with no hope of relief.

Cheer® encourages individuals who are overcome by feelings of hopelessness and helplessness. It restores hope when one has been stretched beyond the limits of endurance. This blend inspires faith that life will work out for the best despite difficulties and setbacks. Cheer® reminds individuals there is so much more to life than the hardship they are experiencing, and to determinedly hold on until they regain the hope and joy they feel they've lost.

INGREDIENTS: Wild Orange, Clove, Star Anise, Lemon Myrtle, Nutmeg, Vanilla, Ginger, Cinnamon

NEGATIVE EMOTIONS: Weighed down, hopeless, joyless, heavyhearted, depleted, helpless

POSITIVE PROPERTIES: Hopeful, comforted, believing, cheerful, uplifted, joyful, determined, restored

SUGGESTED USES:
Aromatic: Inhale from bottle or diffuse.

Topical: Dilute 1-3 drops with carrier oil and apply over heart, on forehead, or wrists.

CITRUS BLISS®
Creativity

Citrus Bliss® acts as a powerful fire starter. It returns motivation and drive when lacking. These oils are wonderful for addressing lethargy, discouragement, despondency, or a low will to live. When the soul has lost its connection to the magic in life, this blend helps restore the spark.

Citrus Bliss® also inspires creativity. Every soul has a need to create. This blend inspires creative expression by reconnecting individuals with their inner child and their natural creative sense. It assists individuals in living abundantly and spontaneously, and encourages play and excitement. Citrus Bliss® can motivate individuals to use their true creative power by letting go of old limitations and insecurities. It takes courage to put oneself out there artistically. Citruses bring color and imagination to one's life. This combination of oils restores confidence in oneself and in one's creations. Citrus Bliss® rekindles the fire of the personality and fills the heart with creativity and joy.

INGREDIENTS: Wild Orange, Lemon, Grapefruit, Mandarin, Bergamot, Tangerine, Clementine, Vanilla, Davana

NEGATIVE EMOTIONS: Stifled creativity or artistic expression, insecure, unmotivated, disengaged, discouraged

POSITIVE PROPERTIES: Invigorated, childlike, creative, motivated, confident expression, spontaneous

SUGGESTED USES:

Aromatic: Inhale from bottle, diffuse, or place drops in hand, rub, and inhale.

Topical: Apply 1-3 drops on wrists or over solar plexus (upper stomach).

CITRUS BLOOM®

New Beginnings

Citrus Bloom is the blend of new beginnings. In each individual's life there is a time when the previous chapter comes to a close and a new one is about to begin. This blend is an ally during the metamorphosis and transition phase—where what is about to emerge still remains unseen. This combination of essential oils is wonderful for clearing stagnant energies which are keeping individuals immobilized. It also encourages them to accept where they have come from and see the necessity of their previous experiences. It reminds that while one can always learn from past mistakes, an abundance of compassion is essential while processing regret.

Citrus Bloom inspires excitement for new possibilities as every new road is an opportunity to discover new parts of the self and embrace adventure. This blend teaches joy in the journey. It invites individuals to live the life they feel called to live and pursue the passions that make them come alive.

Citrus Bloom encourages individuals to really listen to themselves and honor the messages received. Its bright, optimistic energy lifts individuals when they feel within it's time to start anew. It invites them to trust there is purpose in each step they take, and to believe in the promise of each new dawn.

INGREDIENTS: Wild Orange, Grapefruit, Lavender, Roman Chamomile, Magnolia

NEGATIVE EMOTIONS: Stagnant, immobilized, remorseful, guilty, stuck in the past

POSITIVE PROPERTIES:
Metamorphosis, adventurous, excited, joyful, optimistic

SUGGESTED USES:

Aromatic: Inhale from bottle, diffuse, or place drops in hand, rub, and inhale.

Topical: Apply around navel, over the heart, and to the wrists..

CLARYCALM®
Vulnerability

ClaryCalm® encourages warmth in relationships, stabilizes physical and emotional imbalances, and fosters emotional intimacy. It is a perfect blend for supporting pregnancy and child delivery, as it strengthens the mother-child bond. This blend assists women in accepting their maternal instincts and nurturing qualities.

ClaryCalm® assists relationships by teaching individuals to be emotionally open and vulnerable. It eases the fear of rejection and encourages individuals to receive true warmth and love in their relationships. It also encourages feelings of empathy for others by reminding them to stay receptive to the thoughts, feelings, and needs of other people.

This blend works as a powerful emotional stabilizer, especially during menstruation or menopause. It releases emotional tension within the reproductive organs and helps release the expectations of suffering and dread related to the monthly cycle. In short, ClaryCalm® encourages emotional intimacy and vulnerability.

INGREDIENTS: Clary Sage, Lavender, Bergamot, Roman Chamomile, Ylang Ylang, Cedarwood, Geranium, Fennel, Carrot Seed, Palmarosa, Vitex

NEGATIVE EMOTIONS: Invulnerable, guarded, emotionally tense, dread of suffering during menstruation or menopause

POSITIVE PROPERTIES: Vulnerable, receptive, serene, empathetic, nurturing, bonding

SUGGESTED USES:
Aromatic: Inhale from bottle, diffuse, or place drops in hand, rub, and inhale.

Topical: Apply 1-3 drops over sacral chakra (lower stomach) or on wrists.

CONSOLE®

Consolation

This blend of trees and flowers was formulated to assist individuals who are in need of emotional comfort. It soothes emotional pain after periods of extreme stress or trauma. Console® assists individuals who are burdened by loss, grief, or tragedy. When past emotional hurts resurface, Console® can assist in releasing these emotional burdens.

When a storm is raging in one's heart or mind, or when there is no relief from fear, emotional pain, or anxious feelings, Console® can assist individuals in taking the first steps toward healing. It encourages individuals to seek divine intervention so they may experience the ever-present mantle of warmth, love, and consolation. Console® helps ease burdens, assists in experiencing a serene heart and mind, and guides individuals toward emotional rest.

INGREDIENTS: Frankincense, Patchouli, Ylang Ylang, Labdanum, Amyris, Sandalwood, Rose, Osmanthus

NEGATIVE EMOTIONS: Grieving, loss, traumatized, anxious, restless, unsettled, emotional pain, burdened

POSITIVE PROPERTIES: Comforted, content, restful, whole, serene, healing

SUGGESTED USES:

Aromatic: Inhale from bottle, diffuse, or place drops in hand, rub, and inhale.

Topical: Apply 1-3 drops over heart, behind ears, or on wrists.

DDR PRIME®
Transformation

DDR Prime® works emotionally as well as physically with the cycles of life and death and personal transformation. By putting off the old, individuals become free to experience the new—this is transformation. DDR Prime® supports the body's sick or damaged cells to either transition to death, or to transform, repair, and renew. Through the help and support of this blend, individuals can assist their bodies, cells, energy, and emotions in returning to a balanced, healthy, and authentic state.

DDR Prime® is particularly supportive in releasing all types of negative family patterns which are recorded in the body itself (in the DNA). It is especially suited for those who struggle with debilitating circumstances, as it helps to relieve feelings of doubt, disbelief, despair, and burden. It teaches individuals to reclaim their life energy and to believe that change is possible. DDR Prime® supports the process of regaining health and vitality by encouraging release of the old and birth of the new.

INGREDIENTS: Frankincense, Wild Orange, Litsea, Thyme, Clove, Summer Savory, Niaouli, Lemongrass, Tulsi

NEGATIVE EMOTIONS: Debilitated, discouraged, toxic, stuck, burdened by family patterns

POSITIVE PROPERTIES: Repairing, balanced, transforming, rebirth, vitality, healthy, open to change

SUGGESTED USES:
Aromatic: Inhale from bottle, diffuse, or place drops in hand, rub, and inhale.

Topical: Apply 1-3 drops on back of neck or bottom of feet.

Internal: Take 1-2 drops under the tongue, in a capsule, or in water.

DEEP BLUE®
Surrendering Pain

Deep Blue® is generally used for physical discomfort, but it can also assist individuals who are resisting or avoiding the emotions that underlie their physical discomfort. It offers strength to face emotional wounds, allowing the wounds to surface for transformation and healing. This blend can teach individuals how to be the observer of their painful experiences rather than overidentifying with them. When individuals suffer from intense emotional or physical pain, it is common for them to act irrationally or lose their head. Deep Blue® can support the mind in staying cool and collected, regardless of the emotional turmoil or physical pain individuals may be in. In this way, they maintain mental clarity in the face of danger or pain.

At its core, Deep Blue® teaches acceptance and tolerance of pain. It reveals the possibility that pain is not cruel or bad but is simply a teacher. Instead of resisting pain, one may embrace the lessons it has to offer. As individuals let go of resistance, pain lessens and often dissipates altogether. By understanding the nature of pain, this blend encourages an assimilation of all of life's experiences.

INGREDIENTS: Wintergreen, Camphor, Peppermint, Ylang Ylang, Helichrysum, Blue Tansy, Blue Chamomile, Osmanthus

NEGATIVE EMOTIONS: Resisting pain, avoiding emotional issues, panicked, fearful, wounded, unhealed

POSITIVE PROPERTIES: Strengthened, accepting, soothed, serene, healing

SUGGESTED USES:
Aromatic: Inhale from bottle or diffuse.

Topical: Dilute 1-3 drops with carrier oil and massage wherever emotional or physical pain is experienced.

DIGESTZEN®
Assimilation

DigestZen® was formulated to support the body's digestive system. It also has a powerful emotional quality for supporting individuals who lack interest in life and the physical world. They may have a tendency to take on too much at once. This overload of information and stimulation may lead to an emotional form of indigestion, where they cannot break down life experiences into palatable forms. The soul literally becomes overfed and undernourished, as it cannot translate its experiences into a usable form. When individuals are fully overwhelmed and overstimulated, they may lose their appetite for food, life, and the physical world in general. They may become apathetic about their situation and begin neglecting their body's basic needs.

DigestZen® combines powerful oils to support the body and the spirit in assimilating new information and events. It increases the ability to receive new information, new relationships, and new experiences and be open to new possibilities. This blend aids individuals in digesting life's many experiences.

INGREDIENTS: Anise, Peppermint, Ginger, Caraway, Coriander, Tarragon, Fennel

NEGATIVE EMOTIONS: Overstimulated, loss of appetite for food or life, difficulty assimilating new information or experiences, overwhelmed, apathetic, unenthusiastic

POSITIVE PROPERTIES: Assimilating experiences, adjusting, nourished, enthusiastic, engaged

SUGGESTED USES:
Aromatic: Inhale from bottle, diffuse, or place drops in hand, rub, and inhale.
Topical: Apply 1-3 drops over entire stomach.
Internal: Take 1-2 drops under the tongue, in a capsule, or in water.

ELEVATION
Joy

Elevation was formulated to overcome feelings of despair and hopelessness. This blend combines powerful mood-stabilizing oils with joy-filled oils that evoke happiness. The warm vibrations of these oils can soothe the heart and balance the emotions.

Elevation can assist individuals in letting go of lower energy vibrations. Negative habits lose their appeal as an individual shifts into higher levels of consciousness. This blend can raise one's energy levels and energetic vibrations into higher states. It can inspire feelings of cheerfulness, brightness, courage, relaxation, humor, playfulness, and fun. It teaches that worry and fear are not productive, but faith, hope, and determination are. These oils redirect the brain pathways to transform despair into happiness, joy, and abundance. Elevation supports individuals in flowing with life while remaining in peace and light.

INGREDIENTS: Lavandin, Tangerine, Lavender, Amyris, Clary Sage, Sandalwood, Ylang Ylang, Ho Wood, Osmanthus, Lemon, Melissa

NEGATIVE EMOTIONS: Despairing, discouraged, heavyhearted, trapped in low energy

POSITIVE PROPERTIES: Joyful, bright, optimistic, carefree, elevated, cheerful, abundant

SUGGESTED USES:
Aromatic: Inhale from bottle, diffuse, or place drops in hand, rub, and inhale.

Topical: Apply 1-3 drops on forehead, behind ears, or over heart.

FORGIVE®
Forgiving

This blend was formulated to assist individuals who desire to forgive. It is well understood that forgiving others actually sets one free. This blend is especially helpful when individuals feel cynical or begin to expect the worst from other people. Instead of looking for the good in others, they may view them in a negative light. They may also have a tendency to feel justified in blaming others for their own personal situations or misfortunes. Forgive® teaches that everyone is learning and growing together. Mistakes and offenses will happen but should be met with forgiveness and kindness.

Forgive® challenges individuals to let go of bitterness and hostilities and to embrace other people as an extension of themselves, as part of the human family. It reminds individuals to live by the Golden Rule—to treat others the way they themselves would like to be treated. It invites individuals to free themselves by realizing that others are usually doing the best they can and deserve compassion and forgiveness.

INGREDIENTS: Spruce, Bergamot, Juniper Berry, Myrrh, Arborvitae, Nootka Tree, Thyme, Citronella, Niaouli

NEGATIVE EMOTIONS: Unforgiving, critical, judgmental, resentful, cynical, bitter, blaming, angry

POSITIVE PROPERTIES: Forgiving, light, free, loving, understanding, tolerant, empathetic

SUGGESTED USES:
Aromatic: Inhale from bottle or diffuse.

Topical: Dilute 1-3 drops with carrier oil and apply over heart, on neck, wrists, or behind ears.

HARVEST SPICE
Belonging

During challenging times, separation from loved ones and friends is felt more keenly. Harvest Spice fosters the warmth of togetherness and deepens the joy of belonging. Its spicy heat raises the vibration of any space and creates a cozy, welcoming, and reassuring atmosphere. This blend fosters greater gratitude for the people who add richness, kindness, interest, or love to one's life. It reminds individuals not to take for granted the blessing of community, family, and tribe. Too often individuals find themselves separated emotionally, as well as physically, from the people they care about. Harvest Spice's invitation is to create more meaningful connection during time spent together. It encourages individuals to be more present and aware while gathered with the people who matter most.

Harvest Spice is a helpful blend for clearing energetic blocks and overcoming obstacles. Most often it is the self-conscious and unhealed aspects of the individual that create discomfort and strain with others. This blend cultivates a secure sense of self. It assists individuals in navigating the sometimes confusing borders of where they end, and others begin. It teaches balanced interaction where one neither needs to be codependent with others nor distant and withdrawn. It guides individuals to the energetic center point where they can both fully own their life and also freely share it with others. Harvest Spice instills the joy of community and reminds individuals to embrace the sweetness of intimate connection.

INGREDIENTS: Cassia, Clove, Eucalyptus, Cedarwood, Nutmeg, Cinnamon Bark

NEGATIVE EMOTIONS: Withdrawn, disconnected, distracted, blocked

POSITIVE PROPERTIES: Connected, centered, present, grateful, giving

COMPANION OILS: Red Mandarin, Lime, Tangerine, Lemon, Helichrysum, Sunny Citrus, Elevatic

SUGGESTED USES:

Aromatic: Inhale from bottle, diffuse or place drops in hand, rub, and inhale.

Topical: Dilute 1-3 drops with carrie oil and apply around navel, heart, an wrists.

Internal: Apply over the heart and to the soles of the feet.

HD CLEAR®
Accepting Imperfections

HD Clear® was formulated for acne and general skin health. Its major ingredient, Black Cumin seed, is not an essential oil, but has trace amounts of essential oil within it. Black Cumin is prized in many Islamic countries for its healing properties. HD Clear® combines the healing properties of Black Cumin with other essential oils.

HD Clear® emotionally supports those with suppressed anger, guilt, and self-judgment. Individuals in need of this blend may harbor feelings of guilt or anger from the past. These deeply buried feelings may exist outside their conscious awareness. Yet these feelings of pain or anger literally "boil" to the surface. If individuals do not deal with these feelings appropriately, they may manifest through lashing out or blaming others.

This blend supports individuals by increasing self-acceptance and self-love. It assists them in seeing their inherent worth, regardless of physical appearance. It encourages the healthy release and expression of feelings of anger. HD Clear® invites individuals to look past imperfections and to replace self-judgment with self-acceptance.

INGREDIENTS: Black Cumin, Ho Wood, Tea Tree, Litsea, Eucalyptus, Geranium

NEGATIVE EMOTIONS: Emotional pain, angry, self-judgment, concealing, suppressing, blaming

POSITIVE PROPERTIES: Self-acceptance, self-love, worthy, healthy expression, self-aware

SUGGESTED USES:
Aromatic: Inhale from bottle, diffuse, or place drops in hand, rub, and inhale.

Topical: Apply anywhere body needs additional love and approval.

HOLIDAY JOY™
Centered Celebration

Holiday Joy™ invites people to come together and experience the warmth and comfort of positive relationships. It fosters feelings of joy, celebration, and excitement. However, personal memories and experiences of past holidays directly impact how this blend is received. Holiday Joy™ can simultaneously illuminate the rifts, barriers, and unhealed issues carried in families while assisting in the restoration of healthy connections by instilling a desire for togetherness and reconciliation. Coming face-to-face with these realities, compounded by the modern stresses of commercialized holidays, can trigger tension, defensiveness, hypersensitivity, and volatile emotions. This can be especially common during holiday activities with family and close communities. As such, this blend cultivates a spirit of simplification, peace, and connectedness as the focus of the holidays.

Holiday Joy™ can also comfort individuals who are either without family or have estranged relationships due to distance or the inability to heal. While emotionally distancing may be appropriate in some situations where extreme or abusive behaviors are present, this blend reminds that separation is most often not a long-term solution. It offers a gentle reminder to embrace the love and warmth that healthy family relationships can bring.

Additionally, Holiday Joy™ teaches the importance of boundaries in healthy family relationships. This is especially true for individuals who over-give. Oftentimes the desire to please others causes neglect of personal needs and wants. This blend invites individuals to evaluate their motivations of self-validation, compulsion, or guilt. While on the surface this self-sacrifice may seem altruistic, inappropriate giving leads to resentment in both the giver and receiver and is not sustainable. Holiday Joy™ teaches that personal energy conservation and balanced giving, combined with a nurtured sense of self, lead to the healthiest relationships and the most joyful holiday celebrations.

INGREDIENTS: Siberian Fir, Wild Orange, Clove, Cinnamon, Cassia, Douglas Fir, Nutmeg, Vanilla

NEGATIVE EMOTIONS: Stressed, estranged, closed, cold, hypersensitive, defensive, poor boundaries, imbalanced giving

POSITIVE PROPERTIES: Warm, emotionally safe and connected, balanced, joyful, celebratory

SUGGESTED USES:

Aromatic: Inhale from bottle or diffuse.

Environmental: Add several drops into spray bottle and mist around home.

HOLIDAY PEACE®
Contemplation

Holiday Peace® is an incredible partner in contemplation. It captures the natural wintertime state of dormancy which allows vital time for energy conservation and introspection. It reminds that there are seasons and cycles for all living things. The peaceful aroma of this blend invites individuals to surrender to the stillness of the season and allows time to search out the deeper meaning behind their experiences. Oftentimes, reflecting on the wisdom gained from the past will provide the strength and perspective needed for new growth ahead.

Holiday Peace® is also an excellent companion on the journey of generational healing. With its combination of fir oils, Holiday Peace® acts as a powerful facilitator for helping individuals connect to their ancestral story. It gently leads the soul toward truth and discovering what has been unresolved from previous generations.

The body often manifests generational stories held deep within the DNA. Holiday Peace® assists in unearthing what is stored in the body. The body, as a record keeper, stands as a witness to each sorrow, imbalance, strain, neglect, and burden. This blend invites a gentle examination of what the body is manifesting and encourages compassionate listening to the body's messages. It assists the work of restoration, restitution, and releasing.

Although its powerful energy brings buried truth to the surface, Holiday Peace® also provides the gentle steadiness and quiet strength of a peacemaker. It offers reassurance to those being called as the living link to heal the family line for past and future generations and encourages them to make peace within and without.

INGREDIENTS: Siberian Fir, Grapefruit, Douglas Fir, Himalayan Fir, Frankincense, Vetiver

NEGATIVE EMOTIONS: Busy, scattered energy, depleted energy, unresolved generational issues, ignoring the body's messages

POSITIVE PROPERTIES: Contemplative, peaceful, meditative, calm, still, generational healing, restored

SUGGESTED USES:

Aromatic: Inhale from bottle, diffuse, or place drops in hand, rub, and inhale.

Topical: Apply 1-3 drops on legs, bottom of feet, and back.

Environmental: Add several drops into spray bottle and mist around home.

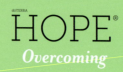

HOPE®
Overcoming

Hope® was blended to bring light into the darkest places. When individuals have fallen into despair and feel there is no reason to carry on living, Hope® reaches out with its reassuring message that there is always a reason to hold on to hope. It encourages the belief that a brighter day will come and helps rally the internal resources needed to keep going.

Hope® combines the healing properties of Bergamot, Ylang Ylang, and Frankincense to address feelings of being unloved, unworthy, abandoned, and filled with shame. It helps overcome emotions associated with lost innocence, stolen childhood, and unthinkable trauma.

Hope® reveals the truth: people are not their story, their pain, or even their experiences. All individuals are beings filled with a light that can never be taken, destroyed, or diminished. This blend reassures that broken things can mend, hearts can heal, and lives can be restored. Through the darkness, its message calls out to hold on, gather strength, and have courage to believe that life matters and there is still a reason to hope.

INGREDIENTS: Bergamot, Ylang Ylang, Frankincense, Vanilla

NEGATIVE EMOTIONS: Despairing, hopeless, unloved, traumatized, shameful

POSITIVE PROPERTIES: Hopeful, courageous, self-acceptance, believing, healing, rebirth

SUGGESTED USES:

Aromatic: Inhale from bottle, diffuse, or place drops in hand, rub, and inhale.

Topical: Apply 1-3 drops over heart, on back of neck, or behind ears.

National Suicide Prevention Lifeline: 1-800-273-8255

National Human Trafficking Hotline: 1-888-373-7888

National Sexual Assault Hotline: 1-800-656-4673

National Domestic Violence Hotline: 1-800-799-7233

IMMORTELLE
Spiritual Insight

Essential oils have been used since antiquity to assist meditation practices, prayer, and spiritual worship. Immortelle combines the power of high vibrational oils with grounding oils to assist the connection between spirit and body, heaven and earth. It encourages positive states of being and supports the development of faith, hope, gratitude, kindness, love, patience, and trust.

Immortelle is a wonderful aid for meditation as it quiets the mind, fosters inner stillness, and encourages spiritual growth. These oils are gentle yet powerful. They assist in the release of negativity, darkness, and limiting perceptions. This blend can mitigate spiritual blindness and other spiritual issues by offering profound light to individuals.

Immortelle offers grace and comfort when one feels discouraged or distressed. This blend can assist individuals in transcending the darkness, pain, and stress of life. It offers support in raising levels of consciousness and preparing individuals for new heights of spiritual transformation.

INGREDIENTS: Frankincense, Sandalwood, Lavender, Myrrh, Helichrysum, Rose, Tulsi

NEGATIVE EMOTIONS: Spiritually disconnected, burdened, discouraged, spiritual blindness, dark night of the soul

POSITIVE PROPERTIES: Hopeful, spiritual transformation, faith, trusting in the Divine, grace, still

SUGGESTED USES:
Aromatic: Inhale from bottle, diffuse, or place drops in hand, rub, and inhale.

Topical: Apply 1-3 drops on crown of head, forehead, wrists, over throat, or heart.

INTUNE®

Presence

In contrast to Lemon, known as "The Oil of Focus," InTune® calms the mind, facilitating inner peace. Whereas Lemon activates the mind, InTune® quiets and grounds mental forces. It is especially beneficial to those with a short attention span. It encourages individuals to remain present with the task at hand and to complete a project, goal, or activity before moving onto the next. InTune® is therefore supportive to individuals who become lost in thought, rapidly jump from one activity or idea to the next, lose themselves in daydreams or fantasy.

InTune® gently guides the soul into full awareness of its physical body and physical surroundings. It invites individuals to accept the reality of their life situation, so they may deal with it appropriately. This blend especially encourages individuals to live in the here and now, and therefore promotes a meditative state. It's stability and grounding energy supports a healthy connection between the body and the mind. With the support of InTune®, individuals are empowered to live fully connected in the present moment.

INGREDIENTS: Amyris, Patchouli, Frankincense, Lime, Ylang Ylang, Sandalwood, Roman Chamomile

NEGATIVE EMOTIONS: Distracted, not present or aware, daydreaming, procrastinating, scattered

POSITIVE PROPERTIES: Focused, completion of projects and tasks, living in the present moment, calm, grounded

SUGGESTED USES:
Aromatic: Inhale from bottle, diffuse, or place drops in hand, rub, and inhale.

Topical: Apply 1-3 drops on temples, wrists, or back of neck.

ISLAND MINT®
dōTERRA
Respite

Island Mint is a delightfully bright blend. The citrus and mint combination elevates both body and mind. When one has felt bombarded by heaviness, recurring stress, or persistent challenges, this blend offers reprieve and a touch of summer for the soul.

Island Mint is balanced by the distinctive depth of Spruce. This oil is especially beneficial for anchoring the emotional lift of the other oils and ensuring that the energy infused does not come at the expense of other vital resources. Everyone needs reinvigoration and renewal at times. This blend provides emotional respite, which inspires individuals to look beneath the surface for the true source of their overwhelm and distress. It teaches that lasting peace and comfort come from doing the necessary emotional work to create personal wholeness. The energetic message of this blend is to balance the very real need to relax and unwind with the less productive impulse to continually escape and avoid the difficulties of life.

Island Mint opens the upper chakras, lifting individual into higher vibratory states. This allows for clearer insight with which to recognize the unconscious fears and limiting beliefs that are holding them back. Releasing these dense elements from the mind and heart allows them to tap into wells of natural enthusiasm and positivity. Island Mint invites all to expand into their full brilliance and rise to meet their life.

INGREDIENTS: Lime, Lemon, Peppermint, Spruce

NEGATIVE EMOTIONS: Overwhelmed, burned out, fatigued, heavy, escapism

POSITIVE PROPERTIES: Relaxed, elevated, reinvigorated, balanced, enthusiastic, positive

SUGGESTED USES:

Aromatic: Inhale from bottle, diffuse, or place drops in hand, rub, and inhale.

Topical: Apply over chest, on shoulders, and neck.

MOTIVATE®
Motivation

This blend of mints and citrus oils was formulated for those who need motivation and encouragement. It assists individuals whose will has stagnated and needs to be fired into action again. Motivate® fosters confidence to follow through with one's creative inspirations and intentions. It also imbues a warrior-like spirit and strengthens individuals to face adversities and challenges.

This blend is especially helpful in times of weariness and discouragement when one has lost the energy and motivation to complete important life tasks, such as caring for a sick loved one or assisting others in need. It is easy to become lethargic or discouraged when one is in a long-term care situation or another emotionally or physically taxing circumstance. Motivate® can act as a support in rediscovering and maintaining one's desire to serve. It encourages individuals to work through their feelings of gloom, weariness, or hopelessness, rather than slipping into despondency or despair. Instead of remaining paralyzed by these feelings, this blend launches individuals into positive action. It confidently reassures that they do have the courage needed to face another day.

INGREDIENTS: Peppermint, Clementine, Coriander, Basil, Yuzu, Melissa, Rosemary, Vanilla, Laurel Leaf

NEGATIVE EMOTIONS: Weary, discouraged, stagnant, gloomy, lacking motivation, unable to press on

POSITIVE PROPERTIES: Motivated, encouraged, hopeful, energized, confident

SUGGESTED USES:
Aromatic: Inhale from bottle or diffuse.

Topical: Dilute 1-3 drops with carrier oil and apply over solar plexus (upper stomach), heart, on wrists, or behind ears.

ON GUARD®
Protection

This combination of oils is generally used to shield individuals from harmful threats. This blend's protective properties, however, extend beyond the physical level by aiding individuals in warding off energetic parasites, domineering personalities, and other negative influences. On Guard® strengthens the immune system, which governs the ability to defend against attacks from both physical and negative energies.

On Guard® is incredibly helpful for strengthening the inner self along with inner resolve to stand up for oneself and live in integrity. This blend is especially indicated for personalities who have a weakened boundary due to some kind of perpetual violation to their personal space. On Guard® gives individuals strength to say no and resolve to maintain clear boundaries. It cuts away unhealthy connections such as codependency, parasitic relationships, or emotional viruses found in negative group thought. On Guard® greatly assists individuals in learning to stand up for themselves and live in integrity with their True Self.

INGREDIENTS: Wild Orange, Clove, Cinnamon, Eucalyptus, Rosemary

NEGATIVE EMOTIONS: Attacked, unprotected, vulnerable, controlled, manipulated, susceptible to peer pressure

POSITIVE PROPERTIES: Healthy boundaries, protected, capable, integrity, independent, reinforced, strengthened

SUGGESTED USES:
Aromatic: Inhale from bottle or diffuse.
Topical: Dilute 1-3 drops with carrier oil and apply over chest, throat, or on bottom of feet.
Environmental: Add several drops into spray bottle and mist around home.
Internal: Take 1-2 drops under the tongue, in a capsule, or in water.

PASSION®
Finding Your Passion

This blend was formulated to assist individuals who are lacking inner passion. It is helpful for those caught in patterns of self-denial or regimentation. Overworking and being too serious can dull one's sensitivity and emotions. When individuals are burdened by a joyless sense of duty, Passion® encourages them to be more playful and spontaneous. It teaches that there is more to living than working and obligation.

When appropriate, Passion® encourages individuals to take risks, to confidently face their fears, and to break free from the limitations they place on themselves. It challenges individuals to use their creativity and imagination to fulfill their life's true desires. In short, when life has become a dull set of routines and obligations, Passion® acts as a reminder to rediscover one's inner passion.

INGREDIENTS: Cardamom, Cinnamon, Ginger, Clove, Sandalwood, Jasmine, Vanilla, Damiana, Laurel Leaf

NEGATIVE EMOTIONS: Self-denial, regimented, duty-bound, serious, dull, joyless, dispassionate

POSITIVE PROPERTIES: Passionate, risk-taking, vitality, inspired, alive, playful, spontaneous, creative

SUGGESTED USES:
Aromatic: Inhale from bottle or diffuse.

Topical: Dilute 1-3 drops with carrier oil and apply over entire stomach, on wrists, or behind ears.

PASTTENSE®
Relief

Generally used to relieve head tension, PastTense® also assists individuals in releasing the stress and emotional tension that may have contributed to or caused their head tension.

PastTense® synergistically combines the powerful relaxation qualities of essential oils to assist and teach the body how to calm and relax. It can also help individuals release the fears that create tension and pain in the body. PastTense® can calm severe stress, soothe trauma, and bring balance to the body and energy system. This blend also helps in regaining equilibrium following periods of overwork, burnout, and fatigue.

As physical and emotional discomforts are relieved, PastTense® fosters feelings of appreciation. It invites balance and reminds individuals there is still much to be grateful for despite opposition, trials, or setbacks.

INGREDIENTS: Wintergreen, Lavender, Peppermint, Frankincense, Cilantro, Marjoram, Roman Chamomile, Basil, Rosemary

NEGATIVE EMOTIONS: Stressed, overworked, nervous, burned out, overwhelmed, fatigued, imbalanced, tense

POSITIVE PROPERTIES: Equilibrium, calm, relaxed, relieved, grateful

SUGGESTED USES:
Aromatic: Inhale from bottle, diffuse, or place drops in hand, rub, and inhale.

Topical: Apply 1-3 drops on head, neck, and shoulders.

PEACE®
Reassurance

This blend was formulated to assist individuals who lack inner peace. People thrive when they feel connected to the Divine. Souls achieve true and lasting peace through connection to this source. Without this true peace, there is a human tendency to try to manufacture peace by controlling one's environment and relationships. Especially when one feels afraid, it is tempting to try to control others because it gives an artificial sense of order and safety.

Peace® invites individuals to connect to the true source of unending peace and let go of control and excess attachments in order to experience the incredible peace that flows from the Divine. It invites individuals to trust in divine goodness and grace. Peace® affirms that no amount of control or effort can fill the empty soul. It reminds individuals that only by connecting to the Divine will they cultivate lasting peace.

INGREDIENTS: Vetiver, Lavender, Ylang Ylang, Frankincense, Clary Sage, Marjoram, Labdanum, Spearmint

NEGATIVE EMOTIONS: Controlling, attached, afraid, spiritually disconnected, unsafe

POSITIVE PROPERTIES: Peaceful, serene, content, still, spiritually connected

SUGGESTED USES:

Aromatic: Inhale from bottle, diffuse, or place drops in hand, rub, and inhale.

Topical: Apply 1-3 drops over heart or throat.

PURIFY
Purification

Purify assists individuals in releasing toxic emotions and entering a cleansing state. It revitalizes the energy system, washing away negative influences. This blend supports individuals who feel trapped by negativity or toxicity. Purify provides freedom from past habits and patterns. It is especially helpful in combating toxic feelings of hate, rage, enmeshment, and in severing other negative attachments.

Like Lemongrass, Purify makes a wonderful space cleanser. It can clear negative energy from the household and the environment, as well as cleanse the air of odor and harmful microorganisms. Diffused in the air, these oils can facilitate emotional breakthroughs. In order to heal, one must receive. But in order to receive, one must first release what is blocking the new, clean energy from entering. Purify supports individuals in constantly releasing the old so they may be open to the new.

INGREDIENTS: Lemon, Siberian Fir, Citronella, Lime, Tea Tree, Cilantro

NEGATIVE EMOTIONS: Trapped, negative, toxic, hateful, raging, controlling

POSITIVE PROPERTIES: Unencumbered, cleansing, purifying, releasing

SUGGESTED USES:
Aromatic: Inhale from bottle, diffuse, or place drops in hand, rub, and inhale.

Topical: Apply 1-3 drops on bottom of feet.

Environmental: Add several drops into spray bottle and mist around home.

RESCUER
Soothing

Rescuer is soothing to body, mind, and heart. This blend restores calm when it has been lost and reassures fears when they seem too overpowering to manage. Rescuer also helps to identify what emotional pain may be hiding within an individual. It helps refine the thought processes so inner chaos can be clarified and emerge into the light of consciousness to be addressed and healed.

Rescuer reminds that pain is a form of communication and often is the result of experiences that have been repressed or sidestepped because they felt too large to deal with. Pain is the body's way of trying to get individuals to see what they have been blocking or running from. At the heart of this behavior is the belief that they will not be able to handle life on own. That somehow they lack an essential element that would enable them to overcome the challenges that beset them. Rescuer teaches this belief simply isn't true. Instead it instructs that there are internal reservoirs of courage and resilience which lay untapped within each person. These qualities can be called upon at any moment when one begins to believe they are there, and they are meant for them to lay hold upon. Rescuer instills the faith that the strength and resources that individuals feel they lack have always been inside, in the deepest aspects of the self, waiting to be found.

INGREDIENTS: Copaiba, Lavender, Spearmint, Zanthoxylum

NEGATIVE EMOTIONS: Unsettled, chaotic, pained, avoiding, overwhelmed, incapable

POSITIVE PROPERTIES: Soothed, quieted, capable, courageous

SUGGESTED USES:

Aromatic: Inhale from bottle, diffuse, or place drops in hand, rub, and inhale..

Topical: Apply over heart, stomach, or on back of neck.

NOTE: As a child grows and moves, they encounter discomfort. Rescuer provides soothing relief and a sense of safety in one's own skin despite the distress that comes when reaching for greater heights and potential.

SERENITY®
Tranquility

Serenity® has a powerful effect on the mind and heart. It is a uniquely calming blend that invites individuals to relinquish feelings of stress, anxiousness, and being overwhelmed. Serenity® can support those who struggle with an overactive mind and inability to unwind. From feelings of responsibility to feelings of worry, Serenity® assists in quieting the mind, releasing agitation, and inviting calm.

When individuals overidentify with responsibilities or fears, they create emotional states that do not support proper rest, relaxation, and rejuvenation. Driven by constant pressures and perceived burdens, individuals struggle to keep up with the demands of their lives. This blend powerfully addresses the underlying states that are often the cause of restlessness, stress, and imbalance.

Serenity® encourages individuals to first reconnect with themselves and discover the peace that lies within, and then reconnect with the humanity in others. It invites them to acknowledge when they feel out of balance and allow time and space for true renewal. It also gently reminds that others are often caught in similar cycles of imbalance and encourages compassion and acceptance of them. Serenity® brings a sense of tranquility that allows space for personal reflection, peace, and healing.

INGREDIENTS: Lavender, Cedarwood, Ho Wood, Ylang Ylang, Marjoram, Roman Chamomile, Vetiver, Vanilla, Sandalwood

NEGATIVE EMOTIONS: Stressed, emotional overload, agitated, restless, anxious, disconnected

POSITIVE PROPERTIES: Calm, tranquil, peaceful, relaxed, compassionate, connected

SUGGESTED USES:
Aromatic: Inhale from bottle, diffuse, or place drops in hand, rub, and inhale.
Topical: Apply 1-3 drops on temples, shoulders, neck, or wrists.

SLIM & SASSY®

Inner Beauty

In addition to supporting the physical aspects of weight management, this blend may also be used to address the emotional patterns which underlie and contribute to weight. Those in need of Slim & Sassy® may set strict standards for themselves in diet or weight-loss programs. They believe that by denying themselves dietary pleasures and controlling their bodies, they will force their desired result. Instead, their punitive withholding is met with whiplash from the body as it desperately seeks to survive. The need for foods and sweets becomes excessive, resulting in swings in diet, weight, and mood. This usually causes discouragement and feeling out of control, as individuals berate themselves with criticism and self-hatred.

Slim & Sassy® can support individuals in releasing the heavy emotions which contribute to physical and emotional pounds. It encourages them to find feelings of self-worth. As they accept their body as it is, the body can more easily move toward its ideal expression. Slim & Sassy® encourages all to rise above self-judgment by embracing the body's natural beauty and inherent value, regardless of weight, shape, or size.

INGREDIENTS: Grapefruit, Lemon, Peppermint, Ginger, Cinnamon

NEGATIVE EMOTIONS: Self-criticism, worthless, disgust or hate for physical appearance, strict, self-judgment, body shame

POSITIVE PROPERTIES: Worthy, self-acceptance, confident, embracing the body's individual beauty

SUGGESTED USES:
Aromatic: Inhale from bottle or diffuse.
Topical: Dilute 1-3 drops with carrier oil and apply anywhere body needs additional love and approval.
Internal: Take 1-2 drops under the tongue, in a capsule, or in water.

STEADY®
Grounding

Steady® offers deeply grounding and centering energy to individuals when they are faced with the unknown. People rarely feel comfortable with circumstances that are out of their control and the outcome is hard to predict. It is all too easy to let anxious anticipation disrupt the natural flow of energy and give into fear or even give up. Steady® encourages individuals to simply keep going forward, holding on to the faith that whatever is supposed to happen will happen, even if they don't understand how. And to trust that someday the path they have been walking will be illuminated.

Beyond times of crisis, the oils in Steady® help the individual feel stable and supported enough to embrace personal introspection and seasons of dedicated healing. This blend also has a nurturing quality that offers refuge from the storm. Within this safe haven, individuals can reflect on what it means to live from their own unique, authentic place inside. Steady® provides strength to help them believe they are capable of beautifully navigating their particular journey through life. Steady® instills the faith that the strength and resources they feel they lack have always been inside, in the deepest aspects of the self, waiting to be found.

INGREDIENTS: Amyris, Balsam Fir, Coriander, Magnolia

NEGATIVE EMOTIONS: Unstable, incapable, out of control, inauthentic

POSITIVE PROPERTIES: Steady, grounded, centered, authentic

SUGGESTED USES:
Aromatic: Inhale from bottle, diffuse, or place drops in hand, rub, and inhale.

Topical: Apply over heart or on bottom of feet.

NOTE: The journey to greater self-control can be a challenge. Children are often ungrounded or even reckless in their actions. Steady® instills confidence to choose better behavior and learn to trust themselves.

STRONGER®

Protective

Stronger® imparts true emotional and physical strength. The concept of strength is oftentimes misconstrued to only include physical endurance, mental determination, stoicism, or other one-dimensional facets. This blend invigorates the body with physical strength when needed and restores it when depleted or weakened. However, it also offers emotional fortification and rejuvenation.

Stronger® helps to shield individuals from the intense emotions of others, protecting them from absorbing the negative emotions—conscious or unconscious—in their communities. While this blend assists with energetic autonomy, it also encourages individuals to learn from people who are examples of positive strength and know how to maintain good boundaries.

Stronger® teaches how to draw strength from the Divine. It urges individuals to model their strength after divine strength, which is based in truth and love. It reminds individuals that inner fortitude grows with self-love and love for others. The deeply resonating message of Stronger® is that when an individual is living from their center of truth, they are at their strongest.

INGREDIENTS: Cedarwood, Litsea, Frankincense, Rose

NEGATIVE EMOTIONS: Weakened, exposed, susceptible, weak boundaries

POSITIVE PROPERTIES: Strengthened, protected, rejuvenated, autonomous, healthy boundaries

SUGGESTED USES:
Aromatic: Inhale from bottle, diffuse, or place drops in hand, rub, and inhale.

Topical: Apply over heart or on bottom of feet.

NOTE: Succumbing to undo pressure, letting down their guard for love or acceptance, or an being unwilling to cooperate with healthy practices can compromise a child's natural immunities. Stronger® is both restoring and preventing and offers a shield of protection for children of all ages.

SUNNY CITRUS
Enjoyment

Sunny Citrus is all about embracing carefree moments. It insists individuals take time to reconnect and remember the childlike part of the soul that is unburdened by the stresses, worries, and seriousness of life. Most adults struggle to let go of the responsibility and demands of their lives even for a short time. This results in a fettered, heavy feeling that can only find an antidote in laughter and play.

When individuals find themselves feeling stagnant, cynical, perfectionistic, apathetic, or stifled, Sunny Citrus invites them to throw off the shackles and embrace the optimism, enthusiasm, and spontaneity of youth. It clearly reminds that creativity needs to be fed with humor, curiosity, and healthy risk. The soul craves new and exhilarating experiences to flourish and shine. This blend invites individuals to embrace the abundance all around them and to believe that they too were meant for lighthearted moments and a simpler existence. The message is simple: it's time to stop stressing and start playing!

INGREDIENTS: Grapefruit, Wild Orange, Peppermint

NEGATIVE EMOTIONS: Stressed, burdened, overly serious and responsible, stagnant, cynical, perfectionistic, stifled

POSITIVE PROPERTIES: Childlike, carefree, playful, optimistic, enthusiastic, spontaneous, sense of humor

SUGGESTED USES:
Aromatic: Inhale from bottle, diffuse, or place drops in hand, rub, and inhale.

Topical: Apply 1-3 drops over solar plexus (upper stomach) or on wrists.

TAMER®
Integration

Tamer® helps individuals integrate their thoughts, feelings, and experiences. The human digestive system is a complex and beautiful system meant to break down and absorb everything an individual is taking into the body. However, due to the gut-brain connection, if an individual is struggling to assimilate feelings, they will often manifest in digestive distress. Tamer® invites individuals to see their symptoms as potential messengers of underlying emotional unease and to take the opportunity to reassess.

Tamer® assists at times when individuals are feeling incongruent or unsure of how to cope with the challenges in their life. It invites them back into their center to uncover emotions that may have been pushed down or suppressed so they can be acknowledged and released. This blend is very helpful not only in seeing what they may have been hiding, but also to gain inner clarity about how they truly feel about a situation. Once clarity is gained, Tamer® is also a motivator for taking action to live in better alignment.

Tamer® offers reprieve when individuals have been absorbing the emotions of others and are unsure of their personal responsibility in managing their own feelings versus the feelings of those around them. This blend asks them to focus on tending to their own feelings and well-being. Tamer® reminds all to trust their instincts and have the confidence to choose what is best for their life.

INGREDIENTS: Spearmint, Japanese Peppermint, Ginger, Parsley Seed, Black Pepper

NEGATIVE EMOTIONS: Incongruent, difficulty assimilating, overwhelmed, unclear, hiding, codependent

SUGGESTED USES:

Aromatic: Inhale from bottle, diffuse, or place drops in hand, rub, and inhale.

Topical: Apply 1-3 drops over stomach or on forehead.

NOTE: The ability to process experiences, break them down, absorb what is worth keeping, and let the rest go isn't always easy for children. Tamer® encourages a willingness to assimilate and be shaped by life's lessons.

> **NOTE:** The Kids Collection was specifically formulated with smaller bodies in mind, with each blend purposely diluted to offer a softer, more gentle experience. These formulations also work well for those with fragile health or skin, or who are highly sensitive. They serve both young and old alike.

TERRASHIELD®
Shielding

TerraShield® was formulated as an insect repellent, but it also offers so much more. This blend helps individuals stay calm in the face of danger or attack. TerraShield® strengthens the protective shield around the body, bringing feelings of safety. This is especially important for children and adults who unconsciously merge with other people's energy. They may do this as a way to relieve others' burdens, or to simply lighten the load in the environment. Regardless of the motives, this type of energetic merging weakens individuals' energy systems. Babies and young children are especially susceptible to trying to carry loved ones' feelings, as they struggle to know which emotions are theirs and which belong to other people. This blend can assist individuals in separating their own energy from another's.

While the confusion between boundaries is often unintentional, there are also those who would target or attack others. TerraShield® teaches individuals to hold strong boundaries and not allow themselves to be pushed around. It imbues individuals with courage and confidence to stand up for themselves and face their attackers.

INGREDIENTS: Ylang Ylang, Tamanu, Nootka, Cedarwood, Catnip, Lemon Eucalyptus, Litsea, Vanilla, Arborvitae

NEGATIVE EMOTIONS: Unprotected, attacked, defenseless, poor boundaries

POSITIVE PROPERTIES: Courageous, confident, self-contained, safe, strong boundaries

SUGGESTED USES:
Aromatic: Inhale from bottle, diffuse, or place drops in hand, rub, and inhale.

Topical: Place 1 drop in hand, rub, and brush over clothes.

Environmental: Add several drops into spray bottle and mist on body or around home.

THINKER®

Focus

Thinker® helps individuals focus amidst a world full of distractions and competing priorities. These days it seems everything is competing for an individual's finite time, attention, and energy. It's all too easy to become overstimulated and struggle to pay attention to an immediate task as the mind is bombarded with information coming from more directions and in more decibels than in any other era of the world. In this state it can be especially hard to transition smoothly between activities—even daily activities—as it often requires a dramatic readjustment to vastly different energies and stimuli. When an individual is having a hard time concentrating or handling transition, Thinker® blend will help promote calm and focus the mind to respond to the task at hand.

Thinker® is particularly beneficial for helping individuals cut out distractions and learn to tell the difference between knowledge that builds them up, and knowledge that is actually tearing them (or other people) down. In other words, how to recognize that which imparts energy to revitalize the soul, or that which steals away precious energy resources. This blend is a remedy for a modern world. It encourages individuals not to be misled, distracted, or overpowered by the cacophony around them. Instead, Thinker® instructs individuals to take responsibility for choosing how to spend each moment, asking them to reprioritize their lives in order to focus on what matters most.

INGREDIENTS: Vetiver, Peppermint, Clementine, and Rosemary

NEGATIVE EMOTIONS: Distracted, inattentive, overstimulated, unfocused

POSITIVE PROPERTIES: Focused, attentive, engaged, mental clarity

SUGGESTED USES:

Aromatic: Inhale from bottle, diffuse, or place drops in hand, rub, and inhale.

Topical: Apply over temples, back of neck, or hand between thumb and forefinger.

NOTE: Knowing what to pay attention to requires the capacity to prioritize what deserves attention. Children are learning how to think for themselves, and Thinker® settles, stimulates, calms, and refreshes the mind.

WHISPER®

Femininity

The benefits of Whisper® are not limited to women alone. While this blend possesses a strong feminine quality, female energy is often needed by both men and women.

Whisper® softens overly masculine individuals by getting them in touch with their feminine side. It encourages letting go of pride and tough exteriors, and allows gentleness and emotional connection. It is also particularly helpful when dealing with issues that manifest as anger, hostility, or resistance toward women.

Whisper® also assists individuals in healing their relationships with their mothers, grandmothers, and other women. It helps them reconnect with their mother when there has been strain, separation, loss, or abuse in the relationship. Both men and women can reject the feminine aspect of sexuality as a result of traumatic experiences. This blend challenges individuals to work through issues relating to femininity and sexuality. If individuals have rejected their feminine energy, isolated from women, or disconnected sexually, this blend invites them to heal wounds and find balance by reconnecting with positive femininity.

INGREDIENTS: Patchouli, Bergamot, Sandalwood, Rose, Vanilla, Jasmine, Cinnamon, Vetiver, Labdanum, Cocoa, Ylang Ylang

NEGATIVE EMOTIONS: Blocked or imbalanced female energy, overly masculine, angry or resistant toward women, women issues, repressed sexuality, disconnected from mother

POSITIVE PROPERTIES: Acceptance of femininity, kind, gentle, connected to mother, healthy sexuality

SUGGESTED USES:
Aromatic: Inhale from bottle, diffuse, or place drops in hand, rub, and inhale.

Topical: Apply 1-3 over sacral chakra (lower stomach) or heart.

ZENDOCRINE®
Vitality & Transition

Zendocrine® was designed to cleanse the organs and systems of the body. Emotionally, this blend assists during times of transition and change. It can assist an individual in detoxing old habits and limiting beliefs. When an individual has felt trapped by self-sabotaging behaviors, Zendocrine® paves the way for new life experiences. It aids in letting go of behaviors that are destructive to health and happiness. It is especially helpful during major life changes which require adjustments in habit and lifestyle, such as altering diet, quitting smoking, or leaving a toxic relationship.

Zendocrine® reawakens vital life energy. It also assists in discovering new energy and vitality by encouraging the release of physical and emotional toxins. This blend aids in shedding apathy and any destructive habit, helping a person find new enthusiasm for life. As individuals let go of limiting beliefs, behaviors, and lifestyles, they have greater room to receive. As a result, they are able to see life from a fresh perspective and embrace new experiences.

INGREDIENTS: Tangerine, Rosemary, Geranium, Juniper Berry, Cilantro

NEGATIVE EMOTIONS: Self-sabotage, difficulty with transitions, toxicity, limiting beliefs, apathetic

POSITIVE PROPERTIES: Ability to adjust, revitalized, purifying, open to new experiences

SUGGESTED USES:
Aromatic: Inhale from bottle, diffuse, or place drops in hand, rub, and inhale.

Topical: Apply 1-3 drops over solar plexus (upper stomach), on middle of back, or bottom of feet.

Internal: Take 1-2 drops under the tongue, in a capsule, or in water.

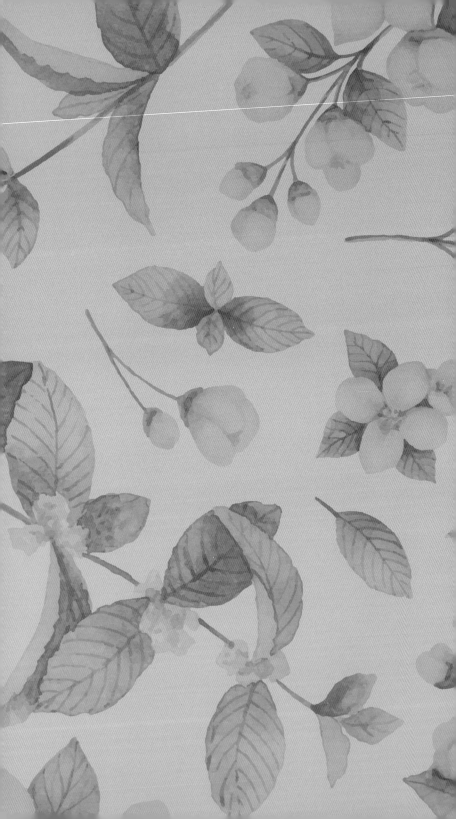

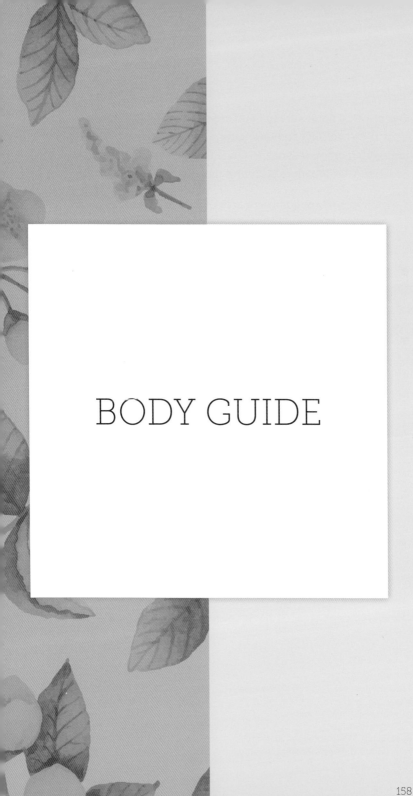

BODY GUIDE

INTRODUCTION

BODY

Our physical bodies are brilliant at providing us with messages to help us be healthier and feel better. Our bodies often reveal deeper underlying emotional needs. Once these emotional needs are addressed, we are more clear and more free.

1. Choose the condition or area of concern that is asking for your attention. If that is not listed, find the related body system or body part.

❀ 2. Read the **Emotional Root** for that body part. Does the description give you more insight into what you might be experiencing? Pay attention to the thoughts that arise.

♥ 3. Review the **Underlying Emotions** listed. If one stands out to you, consider looking it up in the Emotions Guide to find targeted essential oils and processing support.

⇩ 4. **Look Deeper** with questions to access subconscious programming and get to the root of your concern faster. Explore the questions and allow for honest expression of thoughts and feelings, while withholding self-judgment.

This key leads you through the process:

❀ Emotional Root   ♥ Underlying Emotions   ⇩ Look Deeper

Truman, K. (1995). *Feelings Buried Alive Never Die*. St. George, UT.: Olympus Distributing.

Rose, E. (2013). *Metaphysical Anatomy; Your Body is Talking, Are you Listening?*

Hay, L. (2010). *Heal Your Body A-Z*. Oceanhouse Media.

Jensen, W. (2015). *The Healing Questions Guide*. Mesa, AZ: Inspired Body Network, LLC

BODY MAP

The following body parts can be found in this section:

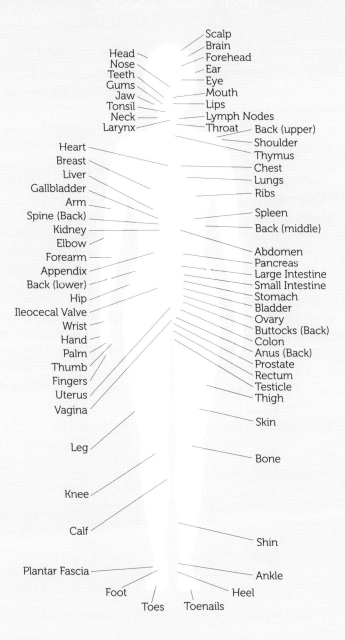

Scalp
Brain
Head — — Forehead
Nose — — Ear
Teeth — — Eye
Gums — — Mouth
Jaw — — Lips
Tonsil — — Lymph Nodes
Neck — — Throat — Back (upper)
Larynx — — Shoulder
Thymus
Heart — — Chest
Breast — — Lungs
Liver — — Ribs
Gallbladder —
Arm — — Spleen
Spine (Back) — — Back (middle)
Kidney —
Elbow —
Forearm — — Abdomen
Appendix — — Pancreas
Back (lower) — — Large Intestine
Hip — — Small Intestine
Ileocecal Valve — — Stomach
Wrist — — Bladder
Hand — — Ovary
Palm — — Buttocks (Back)
Thumb — — Colon
Fingers — — Anus (Back)
Uterus — — Prostate
Vagina — — Rectum
— Testicle
— Thigh

— Skin

Leg —
— Bone

Knee —

Calf —
— Shin

Plantar Fascia — — Ankle
Foot — — Heel
Toes — Toenails

BODY GUIDE

❋ Emotional Root   ♥ Underlying Emotions   ⇩ Look Deeper

A

Abdomen:

❋ Core belief center; beliefs accumulated through experience. There may be untrue core beliefs. Discomfort may reflect social acceptance and how you perceive they are viewed by others.

♥ Anxious, Nervous

⇩ Am I reinforcing positive or negative beliefs with my current thinking? Am I digesting something that is not at home with my current beliefs? What will it take for me to accept myself as I am?

Abdominal Cramps: (see *Abdomen*)

Accidents:

❋ Rebellion toward authority; inability to speak for yourself.

♥ Rebelling, Constricted, Disconnected (physically)

⇩ Is there a pattern of false beliefs that are triggered when accidents happen? What am I willing to let go of to feel worthwhile?

Aches:

❋ Longing to feel loved and held.

♥ Nurtured, Longing

⇩ What will it take to open myself to receiving love? Am I open to accepting myself?

Acne:

❋ Self-acceptance and worthiness of love.

♥ Charitable, Insecure, Jealous, Transforming, Worthless

⇩ Do I fear I am unworthy of being loved? Am I open to accepting myself?

Adrenals:

❋ Represents the ability to comply with life as is; may be weakened by feelings of anxiety.

♥ Anxious, Overwhelmed

⇩ Am I refusing to comply with life as it is? Am I trying to control things outside my reach?

Aging Problems:
❀ Holding on to old ways of thinking; resisting change.
♥ Defeated, Reluctant
⇩ Am I open to embracing each moment of life? What will it take to feel I am right where I need to be in life?

Ankle:
❀ Flexibility related to the future. This may reflect conflict issues with mother.
♥ Stubborn, Wounded
⇩ What issues am I not willing to bend on? Am I holding a grudge against my mother?

Anus: (see *Rectum*)

Appetite, Excessive:
❀ The need to feel protected or safe in your surroundings.
♥ Fearful, Judged
⇩ Am I in a place where I feel protection? Do my feelings scare me?

Appetite, Loss of:
❀ Not trusting life; looking over your shoulder.
♥ Fearful, Hopeless
⇩ Will I trust in my intuition and look to a higher source for positive guidance?

Arms:
❀ Reaching out to others; connection or community.
♥ Abandoned, Isolated, Helpless
⇩ Am I connected with others? Am I holding on to things that are not mine?

❀ Emotional Root   ♥ Underlying Emotions   ⇩ Look Deeper

Arteries:
- ✿ Carrying the joy of life.
- ♥ Sad, Holding on to Past, Stuck
- ⇩ Am I resisting the flow of life? What am I trying to control or refusing to acknowledge?

B

Back:
- ✿ Represents feeling supported in life.
- ♥ Abandoned, Controlling, Unsupported
- ⇩ Do I feel like I don't have a solid foundation in my life? Am I feeling unsupported in finances, relationships, etc.?

Back (low):
- ✿ Financial support or having needed resources (time, money, temporal needs).
- ♥ Unsupported, Vulnerable
- ⇩ Do I have worries about money or the lack of financial or other temporal support? Do I believe resources will not show up when they are needed?

Back (lower):
- ✿ Being accepted and valued by others; having enough in regards to finances.
- ♥ Judgmental, Confused, Constricted, Humiliated, Limiting Beliefs
- ⇩ What past blocks, patterns, and trauma am I ready to remove that no longer serve me? Am I ready to let go of the notion that I have to work for love, affection, and acceptance? Am I ready to let go of scarcity thinking?

Back (middle):
- ✿ Support from people and relationships in life.
- ♥ Abandoned, Insecure, Sad, Self-Acceptance, Unforgiving, Unsupported
- ⇩ Am I running faster than I am able in order to secure the good opinions of others and be enough myself? Am I taking time to self-nurture?

Back (upper):
- ✿ Support in handling life experiences/events.
- ♥ Controlling, Constricted, Humiliated
- ⇩ Do I feel capable of the task before me? Am I making the task larger than it needs to be? Am I carrying more than is needful?

Back of the Body:
- ✿ Past experiences; the private or hidden parts of the self, not available for public view.
- ♥ Angry, Fearful, Insecure, Vulnerable
- ⇩ Is there something in my past that is weighing me down? Am I working hard to hide what I don't want others to see? Do I have things in my past that I don't want to deal with?

Balance, Loss of:
- ✿ Not feeling rooted or grounded in your current situation.
- ♥ Powerless, Scattered, Unclear
- ⇩ What will it take to feel secure in my life? What will it take to trust that life is working out for my greatest good? Do I have a foundation of support?

Baldness:
- ✿ Feeling approval of self. Accepting change.
- ♥ Fearful, Controlling, Unsafe, Holding Back
- ⇩ What will it take to trust the process of life? What will it take to accept myself?

Bed-wetting:
- ✿ Not feeling comfortable about a parent, usually the father.
- ♥ Fearful, Approval (need for), Unsupported
- ⇩ What will it take to feel safe at home? What will it take to dismiss demands that I feel others have placed on me?

Belching:
- ✿ Gulping life too quickly.
- ♥ Fearful, Lost, Worried, Anxious
- ⇩ What will it take to create enough space for each activity in my life? What am I afraid that I will miss out on?

✿ Emotional Root　　♥ Underlying Emotions　　⇩ Look Deeper

Bites:
- ❁ Feeling under attack verbally or physically.
- ♥ Shameful, Guilty, Humiliated, Purposeless
- ⇩ Who or what causes me to feel disrespected? What is causing tension in my life? What boundaries am I fighting for in my life?

Blackheads:
- ❁ Small outbursts of trapped emotions.
- ♥ Angry, Frustrated, Guarded, Argumentative
- ⇩ What will it take to feel safe in sharing my feelings? What concern needs to be expressed?

Bladder:
- ❁ Storage area for anger regarding life circumstances or experiences. Feeling taken for granted or slighted by people in authority and feeling helpless in changing the circumstances around you.
- ♥ Bitter, Helpless, Violated
- ⇩ Am I holding on to deep resentments? What can I do to act rather than be acted upon?

Blisters:
- ❁ Lack of emotional protection. Making things hard for yourself.
- ♥ Disappointed, Frustrated, Annoyed, Resisting
- ⇩ What stops me from expressing irritation or anger? Am I open to creating safe boundaries, even if it means saying no?

Bloating:
- ❁ Ability to process all that is happening in life; conflicted feelings of value and worth.
- ♥ Self (weak sense of), Unteachable, Worried
- ⇩ Am I feeling overwhelmed with all that is happening in my life? Am I self-protecting from an unfavorable outcome?

Body Odor:
- ❁ Not accepting yourself; afraid of others.
- ♥ Alienated, Fearful, Hopeless, Unsupported
- ⇩ What does my inner voice need to express? Am I open to accepting others in my circle?

Bone Marrow:
- ❀ Feeling support and protected throughout life.
- ♥ Unprotected, Unsafe, Unsupported
- ⇩ What experiences left me feeling as if I have been thrown in the deep end? What steps do I need to take to feel like I belong?

Bones:
- ❀ Represents foundational support to healthy body function.
- ♥ Betrayed, Bitter, Unsupported, Whole
- ⇩ Is there a part of my life that is out of harmony with my goals? Is it OK for my life journey to look different than someone else's?

Bowel:
- ❀ Stuffing away negative emotions; focused on perfection. Release of old habits.
- ♥ Anxious, Fearful, Sad, Traumatized
- ⇩ Am I open to letting go of old hurts? What situation am I trying to control to feel safe? Am I open to creating a balance between discipline and unconditional love?

Brain:
- ❀ Represents the conscious director of the body.
- ♥ Distracted, Stuck, Unfocused, overanalyzing
- ⇩ What will it take for me to feel I am the operator of my mind? Am I ready to choose my thoughts rather than have my thoughts run me? Am I overanalyzing things?

Breast:
- ❀ Nurturing others and the self.
- ♥ Overwhelmed, Self-Acceptance, Worthy
- ⇩ Am I taking the time I need to nurture myself? Are the needs of others a higher priority than my own?

Breathing:
- ❀ Feeling safe in life.
- ♥ Self (weak sense of), Fearful, Safe
- ⇩ What do I fear? Am I living in the present moment or fixated on the past or future?

❀ Emotional Root   ♥ Underlying Emotions   ⇩ Look Deeper

Buttocks:
- ✿ Power to act.
- ♥ Frightful, Purposeless, Unteachable, Distrusting
- ⇩ Do I feel able to use my energy and capacity to create good? Am I open to the possibility of things working out differently than I originally thought?

C

Calf:
- ✿ Taking action; optimism in the future.
- ♥ Helpless, Self-Sabotaging, Worried
- ⇩ What is preventing me from moving forward with hope in my future? Do I feel freedom to move around physically and mentally? Do I feel cramped in my style?

Calluses:
- ✿ Hardened concepts and ideas. Overly responsible for loved ones.
- ♥ Hardhearted, Rejection, Burdened, Clingy
- ⇩ What will it take to experience new ideas and ways of doing things? Am I taking on more responsibility than is mine? Do I see life as drudgery?

Car Sickness:
- ✿ Being trapped or out of control.
- ♥ Blocked, Constricted, Fearful, Helpless, Out of Control
- ⇩ What will it take to see life as an adventure rather than an ordeal to be managed? What will it take for me to enjoy the here and now?

Cellulite:
- ✿ Stored self-punishment.
- ♥ Angry, Frustrated, Guilty, Powerless, Shameful
- ⇩ Why am I punishing myself? What will it take to love and accept myself? Am I ready to release the past?

Chest:
- ✿ Expressing inner beauty and love.
- ♥ Angry, Anxious, Grieving, Panicked, Sad
- ⇩ How can I create peace in the grief I am feeling? If my chest had a voice, what would it say?

Chills:
- ❀ Desire to retreat and feel left alone; pulling away from the outside world.
- ♥ Lonely, Avoiding, Reluctant, Unloved, Unprotected
- ⇩ What will it take for me to feel safe and secure? What is threatening me?

Colon:
- ❀ Deep-seated beliefs about the self and life.
- ♥ Distrusting, Indecisive, Insecure, Shock, Unworthy
- ⇩ Do I speak to myself with negative or degrading words? Do I have toxic emotions or beliefs about myself and life that are ready to be brought to my attention?

Consciousness, Higher:
- ❀ Center of innate instincts or developed awareness; personal and spiritual development.
- ♥ Disengaged, Scattered, Unforgiving
- ⇩ What will it take for me to let go of resisting life? What will it take for me to trust and follow my inner voice?

Corns: (see *Calluses*)

Cramps:
- ❀ Feeling obligated to work hard before enjoying life.
- ♥ Guilty, Humiliated, Panicked, Shameful
- ⇩ Am I safe to enjoy life now? Do I have permission to nurture myself?

Crying:
- ❀ Releasing expressions that words cannot be found for.
- ♥ Anxious, Fearful, Sad
- ⇩ Why am I not loving and approving of myself? Can I feel peace in my surroundings?

Cuts:
- ❀ Feeling the need to disconnect from what is happening in life; feeling unwanted or unvalued.
- ♥ Angry, Betrayed, Hopeless, Violated
- ⇩ Am I open to trust in a Higher Power to guide me in my life? What steps am I willing to take to create happiness and self-worth?

❀ Emotional Root   ♥ Underlying Emotions   ⇩ Look Deeper

D

Digestive System:
- ❀ Digesting life experiences; what's "eating" you.
- ♥ Despairing, Despondent, Indecisive, Obsessed
- ⇩ Am I overanalyzing something? What am I struggling to process? Have I discarded the waste I no longer need?

Dizziness:
- ❀ Scattered thinking and uncertainty about decisions; may also reflect feeling and rejecting outside pressures; disconnection in body and mind.
- ♥ Indecisive, Excessive, Distracted, Guarded
- ⇩ What will it take for me to let go of unnecessary details and find solutions for myself? Do I trust myself? Am I ready to claim my power to act?

Dry Mouth:
- ❀ Concern over what is to come into your life.
- ♥ Nervous, Fearful, Closed-Minded
- ⇩ What am I dreading? Do limiting beliefs cloud my perspective of the future?

Duodenum:
- ❀ Social stress, emotional upheaval; connected with the image we portray to others; relationship challenges.
- ♥ Fearful, Unloved, Unsupported
- ⇩ Am I in harmony with my inner voice? What will it take to release comparison and self-judgment from my life?

E

Ears:
- ❀ Accepting truth and hearing what is going on around you.
- ♥ Rejection, Sad, Terrified
- ⇩ Am I not hearing what is going on around me? Am I trying to block something out?

Eating Issues:
- ❀ Feeling less superior to someone close to you; feeling preoccupied

with self-hatred; Attempting to control something in order to feel safe.

- ♥ Blaming Self, Inconsistent, Loss, Rejection, Self-Comparison
- ⇩ What loss can I grieve and let go of? Is there something I am avoiding? Am I open to accepting myself and situations as being worthy and enough?

Elbow:
- ✿ Moving forward in direction; includes relationships.
- ♥ Defensive, Stubborn
- ⇩ Do I feel the need to block out others or protect myself from unhealthy relationships?

Endocrine System:
- ✿ Reflects the capacity to absorb life's events and is also linked to emotional identity. Discomfort may indicate congested energy.
- ♥ Creativity (blocked), Traumatized
- ⇩ What is out of balance in my life? Am I open to receiving mental, emotional, and spiritual clarity? Do I have unprocessed trauma?

Excretory System:
- ✿ Represents body's ability to release the old and unnecessary.
- ♥ Abandoned, Angry, Humiliated, Jealous
- ⇩ What am I holding on to? Do I fear displeasing others?

Exhaustion:
- ✿ Feeling responsibility or ownership for life's burdens; prolonged active survival response.
- ♥ Powerless, Resisting, Unloved, Traumatized
- ⇩ Do I have unprocessed traumas? What will it take to listen to my healthy biological impulses? What will it take to appreciate or value what I do?

Eyes:
- ✿ Represents clear sight and acceptance of what you see.
- ♥ Pessimistic, Purposeless
- ⇩ Am I not accepting what I am seeing? Is what I am looking at clear to me?

✿ Emotional Root   ♥ Underlying Emotions   ⇩ Look Deeper

F

Fatigue, Excessive: (see *Exhaustion*)

Feet:
- ❁ Represents being present and grounded in the here and now; may include feelings of being supported in life.
- ♥ Bitter, Hiding, Rejection
- ⇩ Am I nursing hurt feelings? Am I disconnecting from the present?

Female Reproductive System:
- ❁ Center of creativity and physical security.
- ♥ Insecure, Creativity (blocked), Vulnerable
- ⇩ Is my ability to create stifled in some way? Do I feel stable and secure in my life?

Finger (middle):
- ❁ Feelings toward the self or others.
- ♥ Abandoned, Angry, Rejection, Shameful
- ⇩ Do I know how to express my feelings in a healthy way? Am I taking time to validate my feelings so I can more easily forgive and move forward?

Finger (pinkie):
- ❁ Relationship with authentic health (both physical and mental).
- ♥ Hiding, Helpless, Purposeless
- ⇩ What am I not accepting about the message my health is sending? Am I ready to listen to how I really feel and find healing?

Finger (pointer):
- ❁ Identity of the ego or self.
- ♥ Bitter, Safe, Self-Acceptance, Vulnerable, Worthy
- ⇩ Do I honor myself or think I am enough? Do I trust and value my own ideas, opinions, and identity?

Finger (ring):
- ❁ Relationships with others.
- ♥ Responsible, Distrusting, Vulnerable
- ⇩ Do I need people to "experience" me in a certain way? Do I feel vulnerable in my closest relationships?

© ESSENTIAL EMOTIONS

BODY

Fingers:
- 🏵 Represents the details of life, especially as it relates to feelings of the self. Hiding flaws.
- 💜 Angry, Fearful, Grieving, Unworthy, Worried
- ⇩ Am I feeling peaceful about the details in my life? Am I hiding something in the past or about me that I don't want others to know?

Flatulence: (see *Gassy*)

Forearm:
- 🏵 Protection from forms of attack.
- 💜 Hardened, Insecure, Unworthy, Violated, Worthless
- ⇩ What do I feel I need to protect myself from? What needs to change so that my surroundings serve me? What image or idea am I trying to measure up to?

Forehead:
- 🏵 The perception center; understanding or making sense of what is seen or perceived.
- 💜 Indecisive, Lustful, Pessimistic, Purposeless
- ⇩ Am I perceiving correctly? Is something blocking my ability to recognize truth? Am I conflicted because my intuition and logic are not unified?

Front of the Body:
- 🏵 The future (moving forward); reveals social or public self.
- 💜 Hiding, Insecure, Self-Acceptance, Self-Critical, Vulnerable
- ⇩ Is there something in the way of me moving forward? Is there a disconnect from my public face and my true self?

🏵 Emotional Root   💜 Underlying Emotions   ⇩ Look Deeper

G

Gallbladder:
- ✿ Trusting the good in self, relationships, and life.
- ♥ Blaming Self, Defensive, Indecisive, Constricted, Shock
- ⇩ Am I ready to release grudges I have held onto for a long time? Why am I angry at myself? Do I have shock that has not been fully processed?

Gassy:
- ✿ Not setting boundaries; fear of saying no.
- ♥ Anxious, Fearful, Indecisive, Overwhelmed
- ⇩ Am I not comfortable in setting my boundaries around influential people? How can I respect my boundaries and have others respect them also?

Gums:
- ✿ Moving forward with decisions.
- ♥ Angry, Indecisive, Bitter, Distrusting
- ⇩ Do I trust my own opinions, preferences, and choices? What voices am I listening to that cause me to doubt my decisions?

H

Head:
- ✿ Includes the logic center of the body and the connection to higher inspiration.
- ♥ Confused, Distracted, Indecisive, Self-Punishing
- ⇩ What is my body trying to tell me? How can I nurture myself right now? Are my logic and inspiration in conflict?

Heart:
- ✿ Center of love, intuition, and emotional security.
- ♥ Grieving, Heartbroken, Hopeless, Sad
- ⇩ Am I listening to my heart communication? Is my heart light and free or heavy and in need of rest?

Heel:
- ✿ Fear and hesitancy of moving away from family and family values.
- ♥ Powerless, Violated, Conforming
- ⇩ Am I stepping on others to get my way? Am I feeling stepped on or

as if people "walk all over me"?

Hiccups:
- 🏵 Fear of being on the stage of life.
- 💚 Insecure, Nervous, Bitter, Unworthy
- ⇩ Am I feeling pressure to perform in a different manner? What old habits or patterns am I ready to release and let go of?

Hips:
- 🏵 Momentum in moving forward; feeling safe and supported; hope in the future.
- 💚 Despairing, Indecisive, Stuck, Traumatized, Bitter
- ⇩ What old emotions are my hips holding? Can I invite hope to replace any despair?

Hormones:
- 🏵 Feeling homeostasis.
- 💚 Disconnected (emotionally), Regretful, Stressed, Ungrounded
- ⇩ Do I honor my boundaries? Am I feeling true to myself?

I

Ileocecal Valve:
- 🏵 Crossing the line; setting boundaries, taking care of the self.
- 💚 Neglected, Regretful, Stubborn, Constricted
- ⇩ What is causing me to block my progression of moving forward in life? What secrets am I burying from myself?

Immune System:
- 🏵 Represents integrity within the body; usually a result of how one feels about life and the self.
- 💚 Hopeless, Pessimistic, Resisting, Self-Punishing, Shameful, Unworthy
- ⇩ Have I held deep guilt or self-recrimination? What am I rejecting about myself or my situation? What is causing me to need to escape?

🏵 Emotional Root   💚 Underlying Emotions   ⇩ Look Deeper

J

Jaw:
- ✿ Resolution to move forward; represents your expectations of what to expect in life.
- ♥ Angry, Anxious, Nervous, Powerless, Bitter
- ⇓ Does the foundation of my life feel secure? Do I expect difficulty? Am I guarding or protecting myself in some way?

Joints:
- ✿ Change in direction in life and the ease of movements.
- ♥ Angry, Bitter, Rigid, Stuck
- ⇓ What scares me about change? What will it take to believe that my life is working out for my highest good?

Joints, Stiff:
- ✿ Moving forward; leaving past insecurities behind.
- ♥ Discouraged, Helpless, Failing, Rejection
- ⇓ What part of my life do I need to come to peace with? Am I ready to trust that life is working out for my greatest good? Who or what holds authority over me?

K

Kidneys:
- ✿ Not letting go of negative experiences in life. Bottling up anger toward someone close.
- ♥ Angry, Bitter, Unforgiving
- ⇓ Am I in a toxic relationship? What experiences need processing in order to release?

Knees:
- ✿ Flexibility in moving forward.
- ♥ Blaming Self, Controlling, Negative Habits, Stubborn, Bitter
- ⇓ What am I trying to control?

L

Large Intestine:
- ✿ Center of security with life and your current situation; protection of yourself; addictive behaviors.

♥ Defensive, Grieving, Irritated, Self-Sabotage
⇩ Am I stewing over unresolved issues? What will it take for me to feel empowered in my life?

Learning, Struggling with:
✿ Ability to take in new information physically, mentally, emotionally and spiritually.
♥ Incapable, Helpless, Powerless
⇩ Am I trying to fit into a mold to meet others' expectations? Do I feel safe to be me?

Left Side of the Body:
✿ Past experiences or memories; feminine side of things; relationships.
♥ Hurtful, Rejection, Violated
⇩ What is coming up from my past that is ready to be resolved? Is my nurturing or feminine energy out of balance? Do I have relationships that are being threatened?

Legs:
✿ Moving forward or making changes; may have to do with feeling stable; family relationships.
♥ Fearful, Change (resisting), Panicked, Bitter, Self-Acceptance, Unsupported
⇩ Do I have a past experience with trauma of some form that I have not fully processed through? Do I have unprocessed hurt with my family? Do I feel supported in moving forward?

Lips:
✿ Governing center for the spoken word; trusting your own judgment.
♥ Annoyed, Self (weak sense of), Pessimistic
⇩ Do I see the positive things in life? Do I feel I am able to properly express my thoughts and feelings?

Liver:
✿ The life flow or survival center.
♥ Angry, Bitter, Hardened, Irritated, Impatient
⇩ Do I have bottled up bitterness or resentment that is weakening my zest for life?

✿ Emotional Root   ♥ Underlying Emotions   ⇩ Look Deeper

Lungs:
- ✿ Ability to breath in life; security in taking in all of life's experiences; ability to release emotion.
- ♥ Betrayed, Grieving, Lost, Rejection
- ⇩ Do I feel suffocated by a life event? Am I safe to take in life?

Lymphatic System:
- ✿ Protective and cleansing support.
- ♥ Stubborn, Stuck, Unworthy, Vulnerable, Worried
- ⇩ Are there issues I am afraid of letting go? What traumas am I drawing power from? Is my worry creating a distraction from deeper issues? What will it take for me to no longer feel attacked?

M

Male Reproductive System:
- ✿ Center of creativity and physical security.
- ♥ Creativity (blocked), Insecure, Vulnerable
- ⇩ Is my ability to create stifled in some way? Do I feel stable and secure in my life? Is it safe for me to be a man?

Menopause, Struggling with:
- ✿ Fear of aging and female self-rejection.
- ♥ Shameful, Self-Judgment, Insecure, Fearful
- ⇩ What will it take to accept my acquired wisdom and gifts? How do I accept my feminine changes and love who I am today? What will it take for me to accept a new role in womanhood?

Menstrual Cramps:
- ✿ Engaged in the battle of wills.
- ♥ Angry, Blaming Self, Resisting, Bitter, Shameful
- ⇩ Which aspect of my feminine qualities do I reject or resent? Is there an unresolved issue in my past that reflects judgment or criticism of femininity?

Mental Clarity:
- ✿ Feeling connected in all levels of life; feeling able to accomplish your desires.
- ♥ Confused, Forgetful, Scattered, Clarity (mental)

↧ What is distracting me from focusing and being able to prioritize? Do I have unresolved trauma?

Muscular System:
- ❀ Represents the ability to move in life; the body's ability to defend itself.
- ♥ Controlling, Defensive, Overworked
- ↧ Am I resisting new experiences? Do I feel I must protect myself in some way?

N

Neck:
- ❀ Accepting change; the ability to forgive the self for past mistakes.
- ♥ Angry, Confused, Guilty, Obsessed, Stuck
- ↧ Is there something I need to forgive myself for in order to move forward?

Nerves:
- ❀ Representing communication. Ability to learn in new ways and create new paths.
- ♥ Out of Control, Uncertain, Rigid, Oppressed, Unteachable
- ↧ What will it take to be open to learn new things? Are there lines of communication I am ready to open? How can I be less rigid in my thinking to allow my mind to present the solutions I am seeking?

Nervous System:
- ❀ Center for survival instincts. Affects the ability to connect with the self, others, and the world around. Discomfort may reflect sensitivity to emotional stimuli or protective instincts that are stuck.
- ♥ Overstimulated, Traumatized, Tense, Unbalanced
- ↧ What are my gut instincts trying to tell me? Is my unfulfillment creating the emotion of rebellion? Do I have physical, emotional, or mental trauma that is ready to process and release?

❀ Emotional Root   ♥ Underlying Emotions   ↧ Look Deeper

Nervousness:
- ✿ Not trusting the process of life. Not staying in the present moment.
- ♥ Anxious, Fearful, Impatient, Rigid, Nervous
- ⇩ What will it take for me to trust the process of life? What will it take to feel safe in the world? Am I "living" in the future?

Nightmares:
- ✿ Wishing to fix the worries in your life.
- ♥ Abandoned, Anxious, Fearful, Guilty, Helpless
- ⇩ What is causing me worry? How can I more fully accept all that I have completed? Is there anything about my life circumstances that needs processing?

Nose:
- ✿ Self-awareness and ability to tolerate people and situations.
- ♥ Arrogant, Indecisive, Rejection, Sad
- ⇩ Do I have intolerance toward someone? Am I crying inside? Am I carrying sorrows unseen?

Numbness:
- ✿ Withholding love and consideration. Mentally dead. General lack of emotion.
- ♥ Sad, Despairing, Hopeless, Grieving, Hurtful, Self-Punishing
- ⇩ What has hurt me so badly that I'm unwilling to feel anymore? What value is there in punishing myself? What will it take for me to feel safe to be vulnerable and love myself and others?

O

Ovaries: (see *Female Reproductive System*)

Overeating:
- ✿ Soothing uncomfortable emotions.
- ♥ Unsettled, Hoarding, Defensive
- ⇩ What feelings am I covering up with food? What nurturing does my body, mind, or heart need?

Overweight:
- ✿ Protection of the self; self-rejection.
- ♥ Unsafe, Unsupported, Self-Critical

179   © ESSENTIAL EMOTIONS

⇩ What am I protecting myself from? Am I covering up my feelings with my body? What will it take for me to feel safe with who I am?

P

Palm:
- ✿ Accepting life; being open to receive.
- ♥ Despairing, Self-Acceptance, Distrusting, Unworthy, Nervous
- ⇩ Is there something I need to let go of to make room for new, positive things? What in my life is off balance?

Pancreas:
- ✿ Center for absorbing shock; awareness of personal power to act and the ability to stand on your own.
- ♥ Angry, Betrayed, Defeated, Rejection
- ⇩ Do I feel secure in my environment? Am I feeling challenged in my ability to express what I need to say? What will it take for me to release shock from the past?

Pineal Gland:
- ✿ Connecting to your higher purposes.
- ♥ Rejection, Disconnected (spiritually), Defensive
- ⇩ Do I feel abandoned by my Higher Power? Is there something I fear hearing from the Divine? What am I protecting from?

Postnasal Drip:
- ✿ Internal crying.
- ♥ Violated, Avoiding, Helpless
- ⇩ What is causing me to feel sorry for myself? Am I not allowing myself to feel certain emotions because they are supposedly bad or wrong to feel?

Prostate:
- ✿ Reflection of masculinity.
- ♥ Misunderstood, Defensive, Jealous, Burdened
- ⇩ What will it take to release shame associated with my manhood? Is my sexuality balanced and healthy? What troubles me about my masculinity?

✿ Emotional Root   ♥ Underlying Emotions   ⇩ Look Deeper

R

Rectum:
- ❀ The point of release or letting go.
- ♥ Fearful, Constricted, Blocked, Codependent, Helpless
- ⇩ What am I ready to process and release from my life? Do I feel helpless to my circumstances?

Respiratory System:
- ❀ Center for filtering life.
- ♥ Confused, Defensive, Grieving, Overwhelmed, Sad
- ⇩ Am I keeping life out for fear that I may be hurt? Am I harboring a grief in my life?

Ribs:
- ❀ Having boundaries set; feeling protected.
- ♥ Indecisive, Vulnerable
- ⇩ Am I experiencing healthy boundaries for my higher self?

Right Side of Body:
- ❀ The future; things to come; masculine energy.
- ♥ Apprehensive, Fearful, Worried
- ⇩ What needs to be resolved in me before I can move forward? Is my providing, protecting, or masculine energy out of balance?

Runny Nose:
- ❀ Feeling invaded; needing to protect the self.
- ♥ Abandoned, Hopeless, Controlled
- ⇩ What offense created a sense of mistrust? What circumstances are draining and seem unrewarding?

S

Scalp:
- ❀ Interpretation of how well life is going; rightness in action; itching may indicate transition or feeling stuck.
- ♥ Blaming Self, Self-Acceptance, Unworthy
- ⇩ Am I concerned that I am not doing things the supposed right way? Is there a disconnect between what is and what I perceive should be in my life?

© ESSENTIAL EMOTIONS

Sexual Health:
- ✿ Reflects feelings regarding personal safety and identity.
- ♥ Dishonest, Unsettled, Unloved
- ⇩ Do I have traumas that I am compensating for? What will it take for me to be enough as a woman or a man? What will it take for me to be honest with myself?

Shin:
- ✿ Not feeling in control of how others see and respond to you. Pressure to achieve a certain image.
- ♥ Angry, Bitter, Controlling, Frustrated
- ⇩ What life events feel out of control? Who or what has triggered me to feel angry and resentful?

Shortness of Breath:
- ✿ Coping or processing a suppressed trauma.
- ♥ Overwhelmed, Self-Punishing, Unsupported
- ⇩ What or who in my life is consuming me? Do I have shame, guilt, or trauma that I am ready to process?

Shoulders:
- ✿ Represents the burdens one is carrying.
- ♥ Anxious, Overwhelmed, Overworked
- ⇩ Am I carrying burdens that are not my own? Am I anxious about or protecting myself against the future?

Singing:
- ✿ Connection to the authentic self.
- ♥ Distrusting, Vulnerable, Worthy
- ⇩ Do I consider myself enough? Am I safe to share the authentic me? Do I fear my brilliance?

Sinuses: (see *Nose*)

✿ Emotional Root   ♥ Underlying Emotions   ⇩ Look Deeper

Skeletal System:
- ✿ Represents feeling strength or support in life's decisions.
- ♥ Indecisive, Unsupported
- ⇩ Do I feel supported in life's decisions. Do I feel strong in moving forward?

Skin:
- ✿ Represents outer self or personality.
- ♥ Hopeless, Powerless, Stuck, Violated
- ⇩ Do I feel helpless or believe circumstances are out of my control? What area of the body is being affected? Does that body part have correlation with other underlying emotions?

Sleep:
- ✿ Letting go of the day; moving forward.
- ♥ Angry, Anxious, Grieving, Stressed, Worried
- ⇩ What will it take for me to be at peace with myself? What is my unconscious telling me about pressures of obligations and conditions? Do I trust the process of life?

Small Intestine:
- ✿ Assimilation of life experience.
- ♥ Lost, overanalyzing, Stuck
- ⇩ Am I over-processing the details of life? What will it take for me to trust myself? What is causing me to block my progress in life?

Snoring:
- ✿ Disconnection from physical, mental, and emotional needs.
- ♥ Fearful, Hiding, Unworthy, Vulnerable
- ⇩ Where in my life am I feeling disconnected? What is causing me to feel a lack of motivation? Am I holding on to old patterns?

Spine:
- ✿ Represents feeling supported in life.
- ♥ Abandoned, Controlling, Unsupported
- ⇩ Do I feel like I don't have a solid foundation in my life? Am I feeling unsupported in finances, relationships, etc.?

Spleen:
- ✿ Associated with mental powers; supports metabolism.
- ♥ Anxious, Distrusting, Worried
- ⇩ What am I not processing in my life? Am I empowered to change my thoughts regarding my circumstances?

Stomach:
- ✿ "Library" of gut and intuitive feelings; beliefs shaped by past experiences.
- ♥ Anxious, Fearful, Hopeless, Terrified, Unsupported
- ⇩ What old traumas am I trying to rid myself of? Am I ready to process discord in my life and move forward?

Stubbed Toe: (see *Toes*)

Subconscious:
- ✿ The operator of most actions; autopilot. Must be accessed in order to change faulty beliefs or life patterns.
- ♥ Inferior, Rejection, Sad, Unappreciated
- ⇩ What will it take for me to listen to what my inner voice wants to say? What am I suppressing and don't want to acknowledge?

T

Teeth:
- ✿ Decision making regarding your life course.
- ♥ Indecisive, Overwhelmed, Violated
- ⇩ Do I feel powerless in directing the course of my life? Do I feel indecisive and unable to analyze options and move forward?

Teeth, Grinding:
- ✿ Struggle to trust yourself and safely express emotions.
- ♥ Unprotected, Unsure, Constricted
- ⇩ What will it take for me to release pent-up emotions? Am I safe to express what I feel?

✿ Emotional Root   ♥ Underlying Emotions   ⇩ Look Deeper

Testosterone:
- ❀ The balance between assertiveness and humility; strength and gentleness.
- ♥ Trapped, Prideful, Unworthy
- ⇩ What will it take for me to grab the reigns and fulfill my life's mission? What is causing me to second guess my capacity? Am I aligned with my inner voice?

Testicles: (see *Male Reproductive System*)

Thigh:
- ❀ Personal capability and strength to manifest goals.
- ♥ Victim Mentality, Hiding, Purposeless, Transforming
- ⇩ Am I at a crossroads in my life? Are there past life experiences I need to forgive or release in order to move forward?

Throat & Mouth:
- ❀ Speaking, sharing from within.
- ♥ Disconnected, Insecure, Rejection, Vulnerable
- ⇩ Am I disconnected from myself? What is blocking me from sharing my true feelings? What will it take for me to accept myself as I am?

Thumb:
- ❀ Feelings of self-control; the perceived ability to govern yourself and your life.
- ♥ Failing, Inadequate, Powerless, Rejection, Controlling
- ⇩ Am I holding on too tightly? Am I giving myself permission to succeed? Am I blaming myself or forcing things to happen to make up for these feelings? Would it serve to adjust my expectations?

Thymus:
- ❀ Supports immunity.
- ♥ Attacked, Blaming Self
- ⇩ What is causing me to feel attacked? Do I feel like everything is always my fault? What will it take to stop feeling like the world is against me?

Thyroid:
- ❀ Center of self-acceptance and self-value; ability to control your life.
- ♥ Humiliated, Overwhelmed, Shameful, Unworthy, Powerless
- ⇩ Am I rejecting myself? Do I accept my intrinsic worth and value?

Tight Shoulders:
- ❀ Lack of freedom in life.
- ♥ Stuck, Violated, Overworked
- ⇩ What stops me from expressing firm boundaries? Why do I want to carry other's burdens? Am I ready to live the life I value?

TMJ:
- ❀ Unexpressed opinions and emotions; deeply suppressed feelings.
- ♥ Annoyed, Blaming Self, Frustrated, Guilty, Shameful
- ⇩ Am I comfortable with myself? What do I need to express? What experiences first invited me to feel less-than?

Toe (big):
- ❀ Support and acceptance of life's current direction.
- ♥ Violated, Worried
- ⇩ What is concerning me about moving forward in my current direction? Am I conflicted over changes that may come?

Toe (fourth):
- ❀ Feeling accepted or rejected by loved ones.
- ♥ Hopeless, Bitter, Self-Punishing, Unworthy
- ⇩ How can I express myself to support standing my ground? Am I ready to love me for me?

Toe (little):
- ❀ Safety and security in being vulnerable,.
- ♥ Anxious, Clear, Resolute, Responsible
- ⇩ Do I project positivity about my future self and relationships? Do I feel able to communicate what I want and need?

❀ Emotional Root   ♥ Underlying Emotions   ⇩ Look Deeper

BODY

Toe (second):

- Feelings about the self.
- Inadequate, Self-Punishing
- What steps am I ready to take to move forward in being perfectly supported where I am currently? Am I open to receiving love from a Higher Power?

Toe (third):

- Feelings toward a partner in an intimate relationship.
- Betrayed, Defensive, Abuse
- How can I feel open to receive and accept love from a close relationship? What part of me do I need to forgive?

Toenails:

- Feeling safe to handle the details of life.
- Perfectionistic, Powerless, Scattered
- What will it take for me to let go of perfectionism regarding the details of life? Am I ready to act as the leading character in my life story?

Toes:

- Represents your perceived ability to support and uphold the weight of life.
- Controlling, Fearful, Insecure, Worried
- Am I dwelling on the past, present, or future? Do I believe I can manage all the weighty matters that I am carrying? What concerns me about moving forward?

U

Uterus: (see *Female Reproductive System*)

V

Vagina:

- Acceptance of yourself and your femininity.
- Defensive, Inferior, Hiding
- Do I need to heal from a relationship with my father or other men in my life? Do I feel like women are inferior to men? Do I feel the need to protect from my sexuality?

Veins:
- ❁ Ability to balance and flow with the demands of life.
- ♥ Unsettled, Blocked, Overworked
- ⇩ Do I believe I have more value if I overwork myself? Am I ready to be open to a more positive outlook on life? What will it take for me to be okay with the ups and downs of life?

Vertebrae & Discs:
- ❁ Giving support; taking on responsibility.
- ♥ Bitter, Stuck, Unsupported
- ⇩ Am I carrying the burdens of others? Can I trust I have support outside myself? What is keeping me from feeling safe in my circumstances?

Voice: (see *Throat & Mouth* or *Singing*)

Wrists:
- ❁ Ability to move and act with ease.
- ♥ Bitter, Stubborn
- ⇩ Do I have bottled-up hurt? What hurt am I ready to let go of?

Yawning, Excessive:
- ❁ Represents processing excessive information.
- ♥ Dishonorable, Codependent, Overwhelmed
- ⇩ Am I living life in harmony with my boundaries? What self-nurturing is needed in my life? Am I following my healthy biological impulses?

❁ Emotional Root   ♥ Underlying Emotions   ⇩ Look Deeper

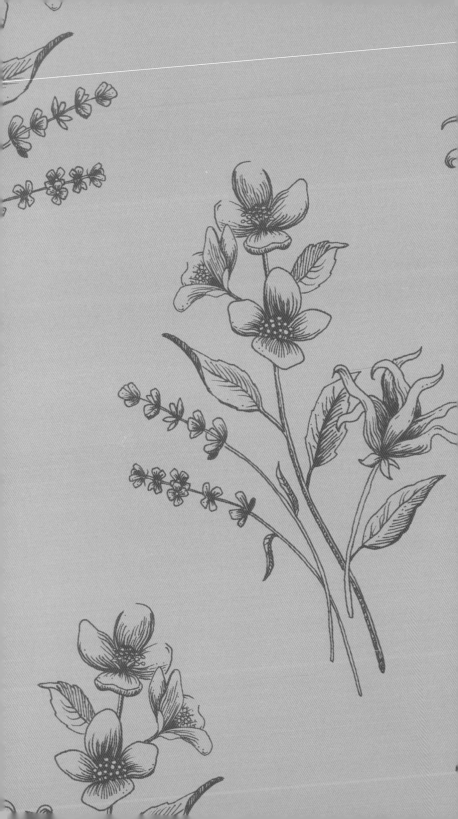

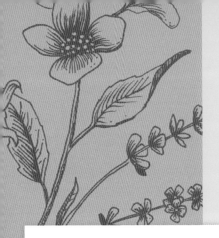

EMOTIONS
GUIDE

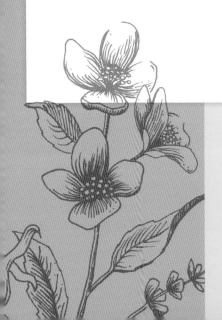

INTRODUCTION

Emotional processing is a simple way to practically apply the powerful emotional support of essential oils. The Emotions Guide can help you process discomfort and feel better emotionally. In this section you will find a list of common emotions, questions to ask to clarify the root of what you are feeling, declarative statements to support subconscious reprogramming, and visualizations to shift biochemistry.

♦ **1. Choose** the emotion you are currently feeling or want to feel. If you are not sure what to name your current discomfort, try looking for what you want to feel. If you need more help, check out the Body Guide. Sometimes it is helpful to use physical discomfort to reveal an underlying emotional need. When you name the emotion you are feeling, the brain emits a soothing neurotransmitter to calm the body.[1]

⇩ **2. Ask** yourself the questions listed in the "Look Deeper" section. Asking targeted questions allows you to access subconscious programming to get to the root of your concern faster. As you ask these questions, allow honest expression and avoid self-judgment for best results. The subconscious mind stores and retrieves your "emotional programming," including habits and patterns of thinking. To pull up the roots of negative thinking, it is key to access this part of your mind.[2]

◀» **3. Declare** the recommended statements to reprogram your subconscious negative beliefs. Use your voice, and declare these out loud. The subconscious mind is obedient when accessed and directed to change.[3]

⊙ **4. Visualize** what is suggested to help shift your body chemistry. Feeling, seeing, or experiencing something in the mind's eye can increase the feel good chemicals produced in the body. The brain can't tell the difference between real and imaginary. The same chemistry is produced regardless of whether your experience is real or imagined.[4]

♦ Oils   ⇩ Look Deeper   ◀» Declare   ⊙ Visualize

1. Siegel, D. (8 December 2014). "*Name It or Tame It.*" The Dalai Lama Center for Peace and Education. https://www.youtube.com/watch?v=ZcDLzppD4Jc)

2. Lipton, B. (2015). *"Is there a way to change subconscious patterns?"* https://www.brucelipton.com/blog/there-way-change-subconscious-patterns)

3. Forsyth, L. (2017). *Repeat After Me; How to Liberate Yourself from the Chains of Mental and Emotional Stress* (pp.13).

4. Hamilton, D. (2014). *Does your brain distinguish real from imaginary?* https://drdavidhamilton.com/does-your-brain-distinguish-real-from-imaginary/

EMOTIONS GUIDE

🌢 Oils   ⬇ Look Deeper   ◀🔊 Declare   ⊙ Visualize

A

Abandoned:
🌢 Frankincense, Myrrh, Marjoram, Geranium, Manuka
⬇ Who or what has left me alone? Do I feel loss over a change in my life?
◀🔊 I am now perfectly supported in every moment. I am now open to trusting and acknowledging that I am well provided for.
⊙ See yourself held in loving arms. Allow comfort and healing to flow into your heart.

Abundant:
🌢 Wild Orange, Spikenard, Citrus Bliss®, Elevation, Tangerine, Cumin, Litsea
⬇ What will it take for me to believe I am worthy and able to receive more? Am I limiting gifts that would otherwise flow to me? Do I have a subconscious belief that life should be hard?
◀🔊 I now allow abundance to flow to me in unexpected and surprising ways. I am now ready and open to receive all good gifts and have permission to do so.
⊙ See yourself open the door of abundance. Notice that everything you need is peacefully present.

Abuse:
🌢 Cinnamon, Clove, Helichrysum, White Fir, Douglas Fir, Jasmine, Turmeric, Beautiful
⬇ What is needed for me to recognize and process boundary violation in my life? Am I open to see the actions of myself and others in the light of truth?
◀🔊 I recognize that I am now worthy and deserving of healthy boundaries for myself and others. I am now open to healing from past abuse.
⊙ See yourself surrounded by a bubble of light. Imagine you can fill this bubble with any colors, feelings, and beauty that is supportive, healing, and uplifting to you.

Acceptance:

- ♦ Rose, Bergamot, Ylang Ylang, Spikenard, Jasmine, Pink Pepper, Amāvī®, Beautiful
- ⬇ What am I afraid of? Do I feel the need to defend against a real or perceived threat?
- ⬧⟩ I am now safe and open to love.
- ⊙ Imagine your muscles releasing tension and your breath becoming slow and even. Imagine what is no longer serving you flowing out of your body.

Accountable: (see *Responsible*)

Actualized:

- ♦ Arise, Litsea, Blue Tansy, Clary Sage, Melissa, Star Anise
- ⬇ What will it take for my dreams to become reality? What am I afraid of risking?
- ⬧⟩ I can now allow my inner desires to direct my outer actions. I am now one in purpose.
- ⊙ See your body, mind, and spirit connect with your higher purposes. Notice the increased potential energy you feel as they are brought into alignment.

Adaptable:

- ♦ Whisper®, Cypress, Siberian Fir
- ⬇ What am I afraid of in this change? What will it take for me to release control and be open to the possibility that I am perfectly provided for in this change? Am I open to different outcomes than I have experienced in the past?
- ⬧⟩ I now have permission to cease fighting against the flow of life. I am now open to trusting and acknowledging that I am being directed for my highest good.
- ⊙ Imagine loosening your grip on a rope. Feel your hands relax as you release control. Imagine that as you release holding on to this rope, the current of a gentle river can carry you exactly where you need to go.

♦ Oils   ⬇ Look Deeper   ⬧⟩ Declare   ⊙ Visualize

Adjusting:
- ◆ Rosemary, Zendocrine®, DigestZen®
- ⬇ What am I afraid of in this change? What will it take for me to release control and open to the possibility that I am perfectly provided for in this change? Am I open to different outcomes than I have experienced in the past?
- ◀ I now give myself permission to take the time and space needed to transition. I can now trust my body and the transition process..
- ☉ Imagine fresh wind blowing new life over you: clearing out the old, dead things and filling your lungs with hope and new life for the future.

Afraid: (see *Fearful*)

Agitated: (see *Irritated*)

Alienated:
- ◆ Birch, Cedarwood, Myrrh
- ⬇ What has caused me to feel outside the group? What will it take for me to create healthy, supportive relationships in my life? What is preventing me from receiving love and acceptance?
- ◀ I now lay down my weapons of protection. It is now important for me to bring value to my relationships.
- ☉ See yourself filled up with divine love. You might imagine this as a color or feeling flowing into or surrounding your body. Feel your muscles release tension and your breathing open.

Aligned:
- ◆ Align, Coriander, Celery Seed, Frankincense, Immortelle, Blue Tansy, Roman Chamomile, Melissa, Tamer®, Tulsi
- ⬇ What will it take for my actions to reflect my inner values, goals, and beliefs? What needs to change in my life so that I am open to Divine direction?
- ◀ I now have permission to allow my inner compass to direct my life's path. It is now aligned with my life's priorities and mission.
- ☉ See your body, mind, and spirit connect with your higher purposes. Notice the increased potential energy you feel as they are brought into alignment.

© ESSENTIAL EMOTIONS

Aloof:

🔹 Marjoram, Balance®, Jasmine, Neroli

⇩ What am I protecting myself from by not engaging with others? What will it take for me to be safe to connect with myself, others, and my environment?

🔊 I now have the permission to be and feel safe in my connections with others. I can now trust that my boundaries will let me know if I need to adjust.

⊙ See yourself filled up with divine love. You might imagine this as a color or feeling flowing into or surrounding your body. Feel your muscles release tension and your breathing open.

Ambitious, Overly:

🔹 Cumin, Arborvitae, Oregano, Amāvī®

⇩ What am I trying to compensate for? What is unfulfilled in me?

🔊 I am now allowed to be enough in this very moment. I now release the need to prove myself.

⊙ See yourself release your grip on control and surrender to acceptance and self-love.

Angry:

🔹 Cardamom, Thyme, Geranium, Ylang Ylang, Spikenard, Siberian Fir, Forgive®, HD Clear®, Turmeric, PastTense®

⇩ What did not go as I planned? What am I afraid of?

🔊 I now have permission to recognize and validate my feelings; I now trust that all things are working together for my greatest good.

⊙ See yourself exchange anger for forgiveness and light. Consider physical movement to release your pent-up energy.

Anguished:

🔹 Helichrysum, Melissa, Copaiba, Turmeric

⇩ What will it take for me to process the pain I experienced? Am I ready to take the next step on my healing journey? What is my body telling me?

🔊 I now have the permission for healing to enter into my life. I am now open to receiving wholeness.

⊙ See yourself filled with light and healing. Listen to your breath. Consider placing your hands on your heart. Forgive®, Cardamom

🔹 Oils   ⇩ Look Deeper   🔊 Declare   ⊙ Visualize

Anxious:
- ♦ Adaptiv®, Basil, Neroli, PastTense®, Console® ᵈᵒᵀᴱᴿᴿᴬ, Serenity® ᵈᵒᵀᴱᴿᴿᴬ, Amāvī®
- ⇩ What do I fear? What do I feel I need to control? Why?
- ◖I now adopt the belief that all things work together for my good.
- ⊙ Imagine peace flowing down over your body. Feel your breath regulate and sync to this rhythmic flow.

Apathetic:
- ♦ Lemongrass, Vetiver, Lime, Zendocrine®, Blue Tansy
- ⇩ What do I fear? What do I feel I need to control? Why?
- ◖I now adopt the belief that all things work together for my good.
- ⊙ Imagine peace flowing down over your body. Feel your breath regulate and sync to this rhythmic flow.

Appetite, Loss of: (see *Eating Issues* in Body Guide)
- ♦ DigestZen®, Fennel

Apprehensive:
- ♦ Cassia, Cinnamon, Melissa, Turmeric
- ⇩ What am I afraid of? What will it take for me to realize I have strength and support beyond myself?
- ◖I am now perfectly supported in every moment. I now move forward in confidence and strength.
- ⊙ See a light turned on in your mind, illuminating what does not belong. Exhale limiting beliefs, and inhale fresh perspective.

Approval, Need for: (see *Inferior*)
- ♦ Bergamot, Beautiful

Approved of: (see *Self-acceptance*)
- ♦ Rose, Bergamot

Argumentative: (see *Defensive*)
- ♦ Lavender, Cardamom, Oregano

Arrogant:
- ♦ Oregano, Pink Pepper
- ⇩ What am I trying to hide? Am I safe to admit that I do not know everything?
- ◖I now have permission to open myself to new ideas and patterns. I can now allow humility to bring strength.

⊙ Imagine a flow of light and knowledge washing false beliefs out of the mind and heart. See the mind and heart comforted in love and acceptance.

Ashamed: (see *Shameful*)

Assertive: (see *Courageous*)
♦ Clove, Black Pepper

Attachments, Negative: (see *Codependent*)
♦ Oregano, Sandalwood, Spikenard, Lemongrass, Lemon Myrtle, Yarrow | Pom, Niaouli

Attacked: (see *Violated*)
♦ On Guard®, TerraShield®, Birch, Yarrow | Pom, Turmeric

Attentive: (see *Distracted*)
♦ Lemon, Thinker®, InTune®

Authentic:
♦ Wild Orange, Cassia, Spearmint, Black Pepper, Steady®, Kumquat, Pink Pepper, Amāvī®
⇩ What will it take for me to stop comparing myself or my life mission with others? Am I safe to express what I think, feel, and desire?
◀ᴉᴗ I now choose to be true to my authentic self.
⊙ See your body as a cluster of circular colors. Take a deep breath and honor the beauty of the colors. Dismiss anything that does not belong in your space.

Avoiding:
♦ Deep Blue®, Vetiver, Helichrysum, Balance®, Juniper Berry, Jasmine, Turmeric
⇩ What will it take for me to confront the discomfort in my situation? What am I protecting through my avoidance?
◀ᴉᴗ I now trust the process of healing. I am now open to seeing the truth.
⊙ See yourself as a tree with roots anchored in rich, nourishing soil, receiving everything needed to be safely present in life.

♦ Oils   ⇩ Look Deeper   ◀ᴉᴗ Declare   ⊙ Visualize

EMOTIONS

B

Balanced:
- 💧 Petitgrain, Patchouli, AromaTouch®, DDR Prime®, Holiday Joy™, Hinoki, Anchor, Amāvī®, Tulsi, Island Mint®
- ⬇ Am I processing an emotional or triggering experience? Am I listening to my inner voice and living consistently with what serves me best?
- 🔊 I am now allowed to listen to and follow my inner voice. This guides me to what is right for me.
- ⊙ Imagine identifying and sending gratitude to your inner voice. See light and love steady and comfort your mind, heart, and body.

Barriers, Emotional: (see *Defensive*)
- 💧 Marjoram, ClaryCalm®, Rose

Believing: (see *Faith*)

Belittled: (see *Hurtful*)
- 💧 Bergamot, Slim & Sassy®

Belonging:
- 💧 Cedarwood, Marjoram, Magnolia
- ⬇ Have I felt rejected by another? What might be limiting that person from giving the love I seek? What will it take for me to be open to giving and receiving love?
- 🔊 I can now trust that I am embraced and valued.
- ⊙ Imagine a covering of love and reassurance placed around your heart and body.

Bereaved: (see *Grieving*)

Betrayed:
- 💧 Geranium, Rose, Turmeric, Ylang Ylang
- ⬇ Have I taken the time to fully validate and process my hurt? Are my boundaries healthy?
- 🔊 I am now covered in peace and protection. I now allow divine love to be forever by my side.
- ⊙ Imagine a covering of love and reassurance placed around your heart and body.

Bitter:
- Thyme, Forgive®, Neroli
- Who or what has caused me pain? What will it take for me to finally let go of this hurt?
- I can now forgive and let go. I now receive healing and light.
- Imagine removing the bitterness from your mouth. See clean water wash over your head and body, releasing the old and making way for the new.

Blaming Others:
- Ginger, Spikenard, Cardamom, Vetiver, Forgive®, HD Clear®, Neroli
- What is limiting my perspective? Why do I have a need to hold on to this?
- I can now accept full responsibility for my own happiness. I no longer need to blame others.
- See yourself remove blinders from your forehead and eyes. Imagine a shield is removed from over your heart, letting love flow into it.

Blaming Self:
- Bergamot, Clove, Copaiba
- What am I punishing myself for? What do I need to process through so I can forgive and let go of negative thinking?
- I am now allowed to forgive myself and move forward in joy.
- Imagine loosening your grip on a rope. Feel your hands relax as you release control. Allow your arms to receive all the love flowing toward you.

Blocked:
- Cypress, Thyme, Oregano, Litsea, Hinoki, Harvest Spice
- What am I avoiding? What will it take for me to feel confident in moving forward?
- I can now trust my internal compass. I now move forward in confidence and faith.
- See yourself dismiss the conflicting voices on either side. Imagine your eyes and face cleaned, allowing a clear perspective to emerge.

Body Acceptance: (see *Self-acceptance*)
- Grapefruit, Patchouli, Cinnamon, Fennel, DigestZen®, Slim & Sassy®

EMOTIONS

Body Shame: (see *Shameful*)
- 🖤 Patchouli, Grapefruit, Cinnamon, Slim & Sassy®, Jasmine, Beautiful

Body Tension: (see *Muscular System* in Body Guide)
- 🖤 PastTense®, AromaTouch®, Patchouli

Bonding:
- 🖤 Geranium, Marjoram, Myrrh, Cedarwood, ClaryCalm®, Douglas Fir, Magnolia, Niaouli
- ⇩ What will it take for me to be safe in connection? What has taught me that I need to put up a line of defense? Do I have a traumatic experience that needs to be processed?
- 🔊 I am now patient with myself and open to the idea of healthy connections with others.
- ⊙ Imagine fresh wind blowing new life over you: clearing out the old, dead things and filling your lungs with hope and new life for the future.

Bored:
- 🖤 Dill, InTune®, Thinker®
- ⇩ Am I overwhelmed or overstimulated? What is causing me to disconnect from the present?
- 🔊 I can now listen to my biological impulses and give myself permission to rest.
- ⊙ See a weight lifting off your chest, allowing your lungs to expand and receive an abundance of pure oxygen and light. Consider physical movement.

Boundaries:
- 🖤 On Guard®, Tea Tree, Clove, TerraShield®, Stronger®, Oregano, Holiday Joy™, Yarrow | Pom
- ⇩ Are my boundaries strong? What will it take for me to honor my space (mental, physical, emotional) and allow others to stay in their own space? Do I have a healthy understanding of what is and is not okay for me?
- 🔊 I no longer need to allow unwelcome influences into my space. I can now honor my boundaries.
- ⊙ Imagine yourself in a protective bubble that completely covers the space around your body. Allow all needed support to fill the protective space.

Brave: (see *Courageous*)

Buoyant: (see *Joyful*)

Burdened:
- ◆ Ylang Ylang, Black Spruce, Arborvitae, Cypress, Wintergreen, Tangerine, Melissa, Red Mandarin, Manuka, Immortelle, Sunny Citrus, DDR Prime®, Console®, Arise, Turmeric, Anchor, Rescuer
- ⇩ Am I carrying burdens that are not my own? Why am I accepting responsibility for others?
- ◁ⁱⁱ I now take responsibility for myself and my own actions. I can now allow others the beauty of their own growth.
- ⊙ Imagine yourself peeling off all of the burdens attached to you. See light flood in the crown of your head and down through your body.

Burned out (see *Burdened*)
- ◆ Basil, PastTense®, Breathe®, Island Mint®

C

Calm:
- ◆ Lavender, Calmer®, Adaptiv®, Patchouli, Roman Chamomile, Sandalwood, AromaTouch®, Serenity®, PastTense®, Balance®, InTune®, Neroli, Hinoki, Lemon Myrtle, Holiday Peace®, Anchor, Amāvī®, Magnolia
- ⇩ What may be causing me agitation? What is not at harmony in me?
- ◁ⁱⁱ I am now being enveloped with peace and serenity. I now cast off any feelings not serving my state.
- ⊙ Imagine yourself releasing cords of anger, receiving forgiveness and light in return.

Capable:
- ◆ Clove, Cassia, Ginger, On Guard®, Star Anise, Turmeric, Rescuer, Beautiful, Laurel Leaf
- ⇩ What will it take for me to trust myself and my life's path? Why am I concerned with the opinions of others?

◆ Oils   ⇩ Look Deeper   ◁ⁱⁱ Declare   ⊙ Visualize

- ◄๗ I now believe in my ability to move forward. I am now safe, secure, and abounding in grace.
- ⊙ See your feet anchored to a pathway; imagine confidence flowing from the path into your body. Imagine your feet intuitively moving forward.

Cared For:
- ♦ Breathe®, Rose, Manuka, Magnolia
- ⇩ What will it take for me to honor and appreciate myself? Do I have negative self-talk that needs to go?
- ◄๗ I can now value myself enough to take care of myself.
- ⊙ Imagine releasing the weary and worn-out energy from your body. See renewing light flow into your body, mind, and heart.

Carefree:
- ♦ Elevation, Sunny Citrus, Green Mandarin
- ⇩ What emotions are weighing me down? What do I feel responsible for?
- ◄๗ I can now surrender all my cares. I am light and free.
- ⊙ See water wash out the heavy darkness from your body and see sunshine warm your body.

Careless: (see *Apathetic*)

Centered:
- ♦ Vetiver, Roman Chamomile, Hinoki, Align, Steady®, Amāvī®, Harvest Spice®
- ⇩ Who or what is my conflict with? How am I out of integrity within myself?
- ◄๗ I am now at peace with myself.
- ⊙ See yourself as a tree with roots anchored in dark, nourishing soil, receiving everything needed to be safely sustained.

Chain-breaking: (see *Change, Resisting*)
- ♦ Petitgrain, Amāvī®

Change, resisting:
- ♦ Cilantro, Blue Tansy, Zendocrine®
- ⇩ What life experience has taught me it is unsafe to try new things? Am I open to ideas outside of my box? What one step can I take today to move toward achieving my goals?

◀ I now release all fear. I am now allowed and determined to do things differently. I also have unseen support at every turn.

⊙ See yourself receive new vision, which illuminates things unseen and allows your mind to be filled with new ideas. Consider engaging in physical activity.

Chaotic: (see *Scattered*)

♦ Lemon, Vetiver, Lemon Myrtle, Rescuer, Holiday Peace®, Turmeric

Charitable:

♦ Wild Orange, Spikenard, Rose

⇩ Is it possible that I can be successful while another is also successful? Do I feel loved and accepted?

◀ I am now filled with charity. I now choose to see the best in others.

⊙ See yourself removing a blindfold from your eyes, revealing yourself and others in their best light. See charity and gratitude flowing through your body toward all others on your path.

Cheerful:

♦ Tangerine, Lime, Wild Orange, Citrus Bliss®, Elevation, Cheer®, Green Mandarin

⇩ What is causing me to feel empty? Am I trying to fill this emptiness with that which does not satisfy? What is the true source for filling this emptiness?

◀ I am now open to seeing the good in my life. I now receive gratitude.

⊙ See heavenly friends pouring love and comfort into your body, reminding you of your heavenly home and the abundant support which surrounds you.

Childish: (see *Immature*)

Childlike:

♦ Ylang Ylang, Citrus Bliss®, Geranium, Wild Orange, Tangerine, Sunny Citrus, Red Mandarin, Green Mandarin

⇩ What life experiences have caused me to limit myself? Do I have unprocessed trauma or shock to release?

◀ I now have permission to be kind to myself. I can now open myself to infinite possibilities.

♦ Oils   ⇩ Look Deeper   ◀ Declare   ⊙ Visualize

EMOTIONS

⊙ See yourself release any cords preventing you from moving forward. Imagine wind carrying you forward to new discoveries, adventures, and learning.

Clarity, Emotional: (see *Clarity, Mental*)

♦ Amāvī®, Clary Sage, Lemon Myrtle, Frankincense

Clarity, Mental:

♦ Lemon, Rosemary, Spearmint, Dill, Peppermint, Balance®, Deep Blue®, InTune®, Lemon Myrtle, Magnolia, Beautiful, Align

⇩ What is the source of my conflicting thoughts? Am I in integrity with my inner voice?

◁ⁱ⁾ I am now clear and aligned with what I know to be right.

⊙ Visualize light flowing from the crown of your head and out from your eyes to see things as they really are. Imagine this light flowing over your brain, heart, and gut.

Clarity, Spiritual: (see *Clarity, Mental*)

♦ Clary Sage, Frankincense, Sandalwood, Lemongrass, Copaiba, Tulsi

Cleansing: (see *Purifying*)

♦ Purify, Lemongrass, Bergamot, Frankincense, Zendocrine®, Cilantro, Lemon Myrtle

Clear or Clear-minded: (see *Clarity, Mental*)

♦ Thinker®, Anchor, InTune®, Rosemary, Tamer®, Adaptiv®, Niaouli

Clingy: (see *Insecure*)

♦ Eucalyptus, Ylang Ylang, Cilantro

Closed-minded:

♦ Rosemary, Oregano, Wild Orange, Lemon, DigestZen®, Coriander, Green Mandarin

⇩ (See *Defensive*)

Closed, Emotionally: (see *Defensive*)

♦ Breathe®, Ylang Ylang, ClaryCalm®, Rose, Geranium, Jasmine, Holiday Joy™

Codependent:

♦ Tea Tree, Clove, On Guard®, Purify, Oregano, Ginger, Jasmine, TerraShield®, Lemon, Eucalyptus, Citronella, Amāvī®, Align, Tamer®

⇩ What will it take for me to allow the person I love to experience healing in their life? Am I limiting their ability to heal by controlling the consequences they experience? What will it take for me to have healthy boundaries?

◀ᴵ⁾ I can now trust the process of healing. I am now allowed and determined to do what is right for me.

⊙ See chains of control release from your body and mind. Imagine stepping into a place of peace and safety where clarity can be received. Listen to your breath.

Comforted:

● Breathe®, AromaTouch®, Geranium, Elevation, PastTense®, Manuka, Console®, Deep Blue®, Cheer®, Siberian Fir, Beautiful, Rescuer

⇩ What did I lose? If it is a person, what did that person bring into my life that blessed me?

◀ᴵ⁾ I can now surrender to healing. I now find a new brightness of hope each day.

⊙ See a weight lifting off your chest, allowing your lungs to expand and receive an abundance of pure oxygen and light.

Committed:

● Ginger, Coriander, Balance®, Blue Tansy, Neroli, Celery Seed

⇩ Who am I trying to please? What is causing me to fear moving forward?

◀ᴵ⁾ I can now trust my internal compass. I now choose to move forward with confidence and faith.

⊙ See yourself dismiss the conflicting voices on either side. See peace settle over your mind, heart, and gut.

Communication:

● Lavender, Spearmint

⇩ Am I disconnected from myself? What is blocking me from sharing my true feelings? What will it take for me to accept myself as I am?

◀ᴵ⁾ I am now held in safety and protection. I now believe that I am constantly inspired with direction for my life.

⊙ See a blanket of peace placed around your body. Imagine its presence allows trust and calm to absorb into the soul.

● Oils ⇩ Look Deeper ◀ᴵ⁾ Declare ⊙ Visualize

Comparing: (see *Self-comparison*)

Comparison to Others:
- 🜄 Beautiful, Bergamot
- ⇩ What will it take for me to accept that I am on equal footing with those around me? Why am I concerned with the opinions of others?
- 🔊 I was born whole and complete, perfectly designed by my Higher Power.
- ⊙ See yourself dismiss those voices or beliefs that feel heavy and wrong. Allow your mind, heart, and gut to be flooded with light.

Compassionate:
- 🜄 Rose, Serenity®, Geranium, Magnolia
- ⇩ Am I protecting myself from others? What will it take for me to believe that there is more than enough love to go around?
- 🔊 I can now release all sorrow and replace it with love and gratitude. I now have permission to move forward.
- ⊙ Imagine healing hands placed over your heart. Feel pure love renewing your heart and extending out to others.

Competitive:
- 🜄 Oregano, Cumin, Pink Pepper
- ⇩ What do I need to prove to myself or others? What will it take for me to enjoy life without constant comparisons? Are there other ways to define winning or success in life?
- 🔊 I am now winning my own game of life. I now no longer need to compete with others to prove my worth.
- ⊙ See yourself discard the scorecard of your performance. Walk forward and notice how it feels to be light and free.

Composed:
- 🜄 Patchouli, Deep Blue®, Hinoki
- ⇩ What will it take for me to trust my inner voice? What is clamoring for my attention?
- 🔊 I am now whole, complete, and anchored to my divine path.
- ⊙ See your breath connecting your mind, heart, and gut. Imagine this oxygenation flowing to the feet, anchoring the self to the present moment.

© ESSENTIAL EMOTIONS

Confident:

- ♦ Bergamot, Cassia, Roman Chamomile, Spearmint, Lavender, Citrus Bliss®, Patchouli, TerraShield®, Slim & Sassy®, Motivate®, Star Anise, Turmeric, Beautiful, Adaptiv®, Davana, Laurel Leaf
- ⇩ Why am I concerned with the opinions of others?
- ◀ I now believe in my ability to move forward. I now have permission to accept gifts, feeling safe, secure, and abounding in grace.
- ⊙ See yourself wrapped in a blanket of comfort. Imagine confidence absorbing into your body through the bottom of your feet. Feel your feet intuitively move forward.

Conflicted:

- ♦ Align, Neroli, Coriander, Marjoram, Roman Chamomile, PastTense™, Yarrow | Pom, Adaptiv®
- ⇩ Who or what is my conflict with? How am I out of integrity within myself?
- ◀ I am now clear and aligned with my highest good..
- ⊙ See your breath connecting your mind, heart, and gut. Imagine this oxygenation flowing to the feet, anchoring the self to the present moment.

Conforming:

- ♦ Coriander, Clove, Ginger, Cassia, Beautiful
- ⇩ Do I have clear values and priorities for my life? What will it take for me to honor my values?
- ◀ I am now allowed to be my own, first priority.
- ⊙ See your body as a cluster of circular colors. Take a deep breath and honor the beauty of the colors. Dismiss anything that does not belong in your space.

Confused:

- ♦ Clary Sage, Lemon, Peppermint, Rosemary, Lemon Myrtle
- ⇩ Am I listening to voices of doubt and discouragement? Are these voices of truth? Am I aligned with my inner voice?
- ◀ I am now clear and aligned with my highest good.
- ⊙ Visualize light flowing from the crown of your head and out from your eyes to see things as they really are.

♦ Oils   ⇩ Look Deeper   ◀ Declare   ⊙ Visualize

Connected, Emotionally:

- 🌢 Marjoram, Vetiver, Cedarwood, Geranium, Birch, Lime, Ylang Ylang, Whisper®, Holiday Joy™, Harvest Spice
- ⬇ Who or what am I disconnected from? What is preventing me from this connection?
- 🗣 I am now allowed to connect with and listen to my inner voice. I am now safe to connect my body, mind, and heart.
- ⊙ See a network of light connecting your mind, heart, and gut. Listen to your breath.

Connected, Mentally: (see *Clarity, Mental*)

Connected, Physically: (see *Connected, Emotionally*)

- 🌢 Patchouli, Balance®, Jasmine, Magnolia, Harvest Spice

Connected, Spiritually:

- 🌢 Frankincense, Melissa, Roman Chamomile, Sandalwood, Spikenard, Rose, Peace®, Manuka, Yarrow | Pom, Arise
- ⬇ What will it take for me to connect with my Higher Power? What will it take for me to process feelings of shame, guilt, or abandonment?
- 🗣 I am now safe to connect with the Divine. I am beloved and always welcome.
- ⊙ See light connecting the crown of your head to heaven. Imagine the crown opening to allow that light to flood down through you.

Consciousness, Higher:

- 🌢 Sandalwood, Elevation, Helichrysum, Frankincense
- ⬇ What will it take for me to connect with my higher self? What will it take for me to process feelings of shame, guilt, or abandonment?
- 🗣 I am now safe to connect with the inspiration ready for me.
- ⊙ See light connecting the crown of your head to heaven. Imagine the crown opening to allow that light to flood down through your body.

Considerate: (see *Kind*)

- 🌢 Cumin, Forgive®, Considerate

Consoled: (see *Comforted*)

EMOTIONS

Constricted:
- Lavender, Cypress, Breathe®, Cilantro, Rose, Hinoki, Star Anise
- What life experiences have caused me to limit myself? What will it take for me to identify and release limiting beliefs?
- I can now release false notions and limiting expectations for myself and others. I am now allowed to open myself to infinite possibilities.
- See yourself release any cords preventing you from moving forward. Imagine wind carrying you forward to fulfill your life's mission and purposes.

Content: (see *Peaceful*)
- Spikenard, Console®, Peace®

Contentious: (see *Argumentative*)
- Forgive®, Thyme

Controlled: (see *Violated*)
- On Guard®, Clove, Coriander, Ginger

Controlling:
- Cilantro, Purify, Cinnamon, Wintergreen, Cypress, Sandalwood, Slim & Sassy®, Arborvitae, Peace®, Oregano, Adaptiv®
- What am I afraid of? What is preventing me from trusting that all will work out as it should?
- I can now accept that all things work out for my greatest good. I can now trust that this event will help me on my path.
- See yourself lay down the defenses you have been holding on to and step into grace.

Cooperative:
- Cedarwood, Forgive®, Neroli, Cumin, Geranium, Oregano
- What am I defending against? Do I feel the need to prove myself? Where am I searching for approval?
- I am now open to new ideas and patterns. I can now trust that good flows to me.
- Imagine your hands letting go of control. See your body flow with, and navigate around, anything you may encounter on your life's path.

- Oils   Look Deeper   Declare   Visualize

Courageous:

- Brave®, Helichrysum, Birch, Cassia, Clove, Ginger, TerraShield®, Elevation, Juniper Berry, Lime, Spearmint, Black Pepper, Rescuer, Breathe®, Hope®, Yarrow | Pom
- What will it take for me to act on my own thoughts and impressions? Who or what life experience has taught me that I must wait for someone else to lead out? Do I give myself room to make mistakes and learn?
- I am now ready to act on what I know is right.
- Imagine an energizing sensation or color flowing up through your body, invigorating, empowering, and leading you to action.

Creative:

- Wild Orange, Tangerine, Citrus Bliss®, Clary Sage, Passion®, Green Mandarin, Davana
- Am I open to thinking outside of my box? Where can I go to receive inspiration? Have I moved enough physically to clear my mind and heart?
- New ideas now flow naturally and abundantly to me.
- See light pouring from the sacral chakra/reproductive area of your body, bringing gifts and ideas beyond your own.

Creativity, Blocked:

- Citrus Bliss®, Tangerine, Wild Orange, Clary Sage, Green Mandarin, Davana
- When have I been burned in the creative process? Do I trust that this can be used as a gift for my growth?
- I am now ready to move forward in strength and confidence. Ideas now flow to me.
- See light pouring from the sacral chakra/reproductive area of your body, bringing gifts and ideas beyond your own.

Crisis: (see *Panicked*)

- Lavender, Basil, Peppermint, Geranium, Vetiver, Yarrow | Pom

Critical:

- Bergamot, Slim & Sassy®, Thyme, Forgive®
- What will it take for me to let go of my ideas for how everything should be? Am I safe to consider there are many ways to do things right?

- 🔊 I no longer need to expect perfection. I can now accept things the way they are.
- ⊙ See yourself remove blinders from your forehead and eyes. Imagine a protective barrier being removed from your heart, allowing love to flow into it.

Cynical: (See *Pessimistic*)

D

Damaged: (see *Hurtful*)
- 💧 Turmeric, DDR Prime®

Dark Night of the Soul:
- 💧 Melissa, Frankincense, Helichrysum, Immortelle, Hope® ^(doTERRA)
- ⬇ What is causing me to feel empty? Am I trying to fill this emptiness with that which does not satisfy? What is the true source for filling this emptiness?
- 🔊 I am now open to receiving love. I am now ready to be inspired with direction for my life.
- ⊙ Imagine love and comfort pouring into your body, reminding you of the abundant support which surrounds you.

Dark, Fear of: (see *Hurt*)
- 💧 Juniper Berry, Yarrow | Pom

Darkness, Spiritual:
- 💧 Lemongrass, Frankincense, Tea Tree, Clary Sage, Melissa, Elevation, Sandalwood, Yarrow | Pom
- ⬇ What is allowing darkness to enter my life (such as negative thought patterns or practices)? What do I need to change in my life to be more aligned with my Higher Power?
- 🔊 I now cast off all negative or lower vibrational energies and fill myself with light and truth.
- ⊙ Imagine a dark mist or cloud around you being dispelled by light and faith.

💧 Oils   ⬇ Look Deeper   🔊 Declare   ⊙ Visualize

Death, Acceptance of:

💧 Roman Chamomile, Frankincense, Spikenard

⬇ What am I seeking to control about this situation? What needs to be expressed, processed, or understood for me to release my hold on my loved one's life?

🗣 I now surrender all unhealthy attachments preventing others from moving forward.

⊙ See yourself find and release each concern regarding death. Notice the flow of grace returning to you. Listen to your breath and allow emotional release.

Deceived:

💧 Clary Sage, Frankincense

⬇ What wisdom does this experience bring me? What do I see more clearly? What will it take for me to move forward?

🗣 I am now shielded with peace and protection. I can now see clearly.

⊙ Imagine a covering of love and reassurance placed around your heart and body. See the covering illuminate false ideas and restore clarity to your mind and heart.

Decisive:

💧 Lemon, Clove, Lemon Myrtle

⬇ What is causing me to doubt my decisions? Who am I trying to please? What is causing me to fear moving forward?

🗣 I can now trust my inner voice. Direction now flows easily.

⊙ See yourself dismiss the conflicting voices on either side. See your mind illuminated with the knowledge needed to move forward.

Defeated:

💧 Clove, Citrus Bliss®, Eucalyptus, Ginger, Fennel, Green Mandarin, Star Anise

⬇ What did not go as planned? What will it take for me to move forward from this experience? What will it take for me to recognize that this experience does not define me as a person.

🗣 I can now accept that all things work out for my greatest good. I can now trust that this event will help me on my path.

⊙ See yourself release your grasp on ropes you are holding on to, giving them over to your Higher Power and opening yourself to move forward on life's path.

Defenseless: (see *Boundaries*)
- TerraShield®, On Guard®, Yarrow | Pom

Defensive:
- Oregano, Ylang Ylang, Geranium, Holiday Joy™
- What am I protecting myself from? What will it take for me to process the harm I experienced in the past?
- I am now perfectly supported in every moment. I am now open to trusting that I am safe to be me.
- See yourself remove protective gear from your body. Imagine restorative light and love surrounding you.

Defiant: (see *Defensive*)
- Oregano, Ylang Ylang

Degraded: (see *Abuse*)
- Bergamot, Clove, Turmeric*

Dejected: (see *Despairing*)

Denial: (see *Avoiding*)

Dependent: (see *Abuse*)
- Tea Tree, Clove, Ginger, Jasmine, Magnolia

Depleted: (see *Abuse*)
- Basil, Peppermint, Tea Tree, PastTense®, AromaTouch®, Cheer®, Holiday Peace®, Star Anise, Black Spruce

Desire, Lack of: (see *Apathetic*)
- Balance®, Fennel, Black Pepper, Citrus Bliss®, Lemongrass, Jasmine

Despairing:
- Elevation, Melissa, Bergamot, Breathe®, Eucalyptus, Lemongrass, Peppermint, Helichrysum, Lime, Hope®, Siberian Fir
- What do I perceive that I have lost? What voices am I listening to? Are these voices sources of light and good? Do I need to process through a trauma, or am I ready to move forward?
- There is now hope bringing light to my path. Good things are now in store for me.

- Oils   - Look Deeper   - Declare   - Visualize

⊙ Imagine fresh wind blowing new life over you: clearing out the old, dead things and filling your lungs with new hope for the future.

Despondent: (see *Hopeless*)
♦ Lemongrass, Melissa, Eucalyptus, Citrus Bliss®, Vetiver

Determined: (see *Resolute*)
♦ Helichrysum, Lime, Elevation, Cheer® _{dōTERRA}

Dieting, Obsessed with: (see *Obsessed*)
♦ Grapefruit, Bergamot, Zendocrine®, Vetiver, Patchouli, Fennel, Slim & Sassy®, DigestZen®

Discerning: (see *Clarity, Mental*)
♦ Clary Sage, Frankincense, Lemongrass, Litsea, Yarrow | Pom, Citronella,

Disconnected, Emotionally: (see *Connected, Emotionally*)
♦ Thyme, Fennel, Vetiver, Ylang Ylang, Holiday Joy™

Disconnected, Mentally: (see *Clarity, mental*)

Disconnected, Physically: (see *Connected, Emotionally*)
♦ Patchouli, Balance®, Vetiver, Jasmine, Holiday Peace®, Magnolia

Disconnected, Spiritually: (See *Connected, Spiritually*)
♦ Frankincense, Sandalwood, Clary Sage, Rose, Manuka, Immortelle, Peace®, Arise, Harvest Spice

Discontent: (see *Aloof*)
♦ Spikenard, Wild Orange

Discouraged:
♦ Lime, Melissa, Elevation, Wild Orange, Roman Chamomile, Red Mandarin, Immortelle, DDR Prime®, Motivate®, Citrus Bliss®, Green Mandarin
⇩ Why did life events not go my way? Is it possible this new way opens to better things than what I had planned?
◁)) I now choose to believe and receive abundance.
⊙ See a bright beam of light aimed right at your heart, bringing new energy and flow to your body, mind, and spirit.

Disengaged: (see *Aloof*)

🔹 Dill, Citrus Bliss®, Lemon

Disgusted:

🔹 DDR Prime®, Forgive®, Thyme, Wintergreen

⬇ Who or what do I need to forgive to let this go? How was I offended?

◀)) I can now forgive. I now choose beauty and light. I now surround myself with that which uplifts and inspires.

⊙ See darkness lifted off the front of your body. Imagine love flowing over your body, bringing forgiveness and new life.

Disheartened: (see *Heavyhearted*)

Dishonest: (see *Hiding*)

🔹 Black Pepper, Vetiver, Cassia, Lavender, Geranium

Disinterested: (see *Bored*)

🔹 Dill, Fennel

Distant: (see *Scattered*)

🔹 Marjoram, Cedarwood, Jasmine, Birch, Holiday Joy™, Magnolia

Distracted:

🔹 InTune®, Thinker®, Litsea, Lemon, Magnolia, Harvest Spice®

⬇ What am I avoiding? What is causing me to feel overwhelmed?

◀)) I am now present and laser focused. I am now granted vision beyond my own.

⊙ Imagine gray mist lifting from around your head. See a light beam fill your mind and vision.

Distraught:

🔹 Breathe®, Console®, Peace®, Rescuer

⬇ Who or what is my conflict with? How am I out of integrity within myself?

◀)) I am now perfectly supported in every moment. I now surrender all sadness in return for healing and light.

⊙ Imagine yourself standing in a peaceful place, being fed, nourished, and inspired. Listen to your breath.

🔹 Oils   ⬇ Look Deeper   ◀)) Declare   ⊙ Visualize

Distrusting:
- 💧 Geranium, Marjoram, Myrrh, Align, Breathe®, Jasmine, Arborvitae, Turmeric
- ⬇ What am I worrying about? What causes me to feel unsafe? Have I been unpleasantly surprised by life in the past?
- 🔊 I now choose to anchor to truth. I am now confident and safe in this present moment.
- ⊙ Imagine yourself as a tree with roots anchored in rich, nourishing soil, receiving everything you need to be safely sustained..

Dominated: (see *Violated*)
- 💧 Clove, On Guard®, TerraShield®, Ginger, Amāvī®

Doubtful:
- 💧 Sandalwood, Green Mandarin
- ⬇ Who or what do I doubt? Am I ready to release limiting beliefs and move forward in trust?
- 🔊 I now choose to surround myself with that which uplifts and inspires. I can now trust my inner voice of truth.
- ⊙ Imagine light flowing in from the front of your body to dissolve chains of doubt, which fall off your back, feet, and head.

Drained:
- 💧 Juniper Berry, Melissa, Clary Sage
- ⬇ What will it take for me to see myself as worthy or receiving the time, attention, and love I need? Am I acting outside of my boundaries?
- 🔊 I am now cherished, valued, and worthy of love, time, and attention.
- ⊙ See kind hands placed over your heart to hold and heal it. Imagine a renewing of your heart.

Dreaming: (see *Inspired*)
- 💧 Juniper Berry, Melissa, Clary Sage

Drudgery:
- 💧 Roman Chamomile, Coriander, Citrus Bliss®, Fennel, Tangerine, Sunny Citrus, Star Anise
- ⬇ Am I awake to what's happening in my life? Am I satisfied with the status quo? What do I need to give up in order to experience transformation?

⏺)) I can now claim my power to act. I now believe there are good things in store for me.
⊙ See yourself step out of the mud and onto a path of progress. Notice that as you move forward, you shed old, unhelpful patterns and receive new gifts and abilities.

Dull: (see *Bored*)
◆ Citrus Bliss®, Wild Orange, Roman Chamomile, Passion®, Sunny Citrus, Lemon Myrtle

Dumb: (see *Capable*)

Duty-bound: (see *Constricted*)
◆ Tangerine, Petitgrain, Passion®

E

Eating Issues: (see *Eating Issues in* Body Guide; see *Dieting, Obsession with*)

Egotistical: (see *Arrogant*)
◆ Oregano, Pink Pepper, Amāvī®, Magnolia

Elevated:
◆ Elevation, Lime, Melissa, Green Mandarin, Arise
⇩ What false beliefs hold me captive?
⏺)) I now surrender all sadness in return for healing and light.
⊙ Imagine peeling a thick layer of darkness from the back and spine. Imagine sunshine flowing in through the chest and out through the back.

Embarrassed:
◆ Cassia, Jasmine
⇩ What image am I trying to preserve? What will it take for me to realize it is okay to make mistakes?
⏺)) It is now safe for me to learn and make mistakes.
⊙ Imagine yourself removing the embarrassment that was once inside your body. See the roots connected with this idea pulled out completely and replaced with light.

◆ Oils   ⇩ Look Deeper   ⏺)) Declare   ⊙ Visualize

Empathetic: (see *Compassionate*)
- Geranium, Rose, Forgive®, Neroli, ClaryCalm®

Empathetic, Overly: (see *Boundaries*)

Empowered:
- Ginger, Clove, Tea Tree, Star Anise
- What decisions need to be made so that I can move forward? Have I considered divine help?
- I now accept my strength and capabilities to move forward with passion and purpose.
- See a force move through you from behind to propel you forward and upward on your journey. Imagine unseen help lifting you over any obstacles in your way.

Emptiness:
- Vetiver, Sandalwood
- What is causing me to feel empty? Am I trying to fill this emptiness with that which does not satisfy? What is the true source for filling this emptiness?
- I am now open to receiving love. I am now ready to be inspired with direction for my life.
- See love and comfort pouring into your body, reminding you of your heavenly home and the abundant support which surrounds you.

Encouraged:
- Melissa, Lime, Eucalyptus, Elevation, Wild Orange, Motivate®, Green Mandarin
- What am I afraid of? What happened in my past to spark these fears?
- I now choose to believe good things are coming my way.
- See water wash out the heavy darkness from your body and sunshine fill you with strength.

Energized:
- Lime, Basil, Lemon, Zendocrine®, Melissa, Motivate®, Blue Tansy, Star Anise
- What emotions or tasks are weighing me down? Am I out of integrity with myself? What will it take to honor my inner voice?

◀꣭ My future is now exciting and filled with good things. I now embrace adventure because I am perfectly supported in every moment.

⊙ Imagine standing in the sunshine; let the light fill you up with new gifts and energy.

Energy, Lack of: (see *Apathetic*)

◆ Lemon, Peppermint, Wild Orange, Elevation, Citrus Bliss®, Star Anise

Engaged: (see *Connected, Emotionally*)

◆ Dill, Lime, DigestZen®, Magnolia, Thinker®

Enlightened: (see *Manifesting*)

◆ Melissa, Frankincense, Sandalwood, Rosemary, Arise

Enmeshed: (see *Codependent*)

◆ Tea Tree, Clove, On Guard®, Oregano

Enthusiastic: (see *Energized*)

◆ Melissa, DigestZen®, Sunny Citrus, Green Mandarin, Arise, Island Mint®

Envious: (see *Jealous*)

Escapism: (see *Apathetic*)

◆ Vetiver, Patchouli, Balance®, Eucalyptus, Jasmine, Neroli, Island Mint®

Estranged: (see *Connected, Emotionally*)

Exasperated: (see *Agitated*)

◆ Basil, Lavender

Excessive:

◆ Balance®, Sandalwood, Arborvitae, Oregano, Jasmine, Cumin

⇩ What am I covering up or hiding from? What do I feel I need to control?

◀꣭ I can now clear my mind to receive new knowledge and thought. I am now an agent who acts, not one who is acted upon.

⊙ Imagine yourself releasing all the cords holding you back. Allow your inhale to draw in what is needed for healing and exhale what is no longer serving.

◆ Oils ⇩ Look Deeper ◀꣭ Declare ⊙ Visualize

Exhausted:

- 🔹 Basil, Citrus Bliss®, PastTense®, Breathe®, Red Mandarin, Motivate®, Blue Tansy, Star Anise, Black Spruce, Bergamot Mint
- ⬇ What will it take for me to honor my space (mental, physical, emotional) and allow others to stay in their own space? Do I have a healthy understanding of what is and is not okay for me? What will it take for me to assign greater value to my own needs, wants, and ideas?
- 🗣 I am now cherished, valued, and worthy of love, time, and attention.
- ⊙ See kind hands placed over your heart to hold and heal it. Imagine a renewing of your heart.

Expressive:

- 🔹 Lavender, Spearmint, HD Clear®, Citrus Bliss®, Magnolia
- ⬇ What will it take for me to feel safe to share my thoughts, opinions, and feelings? What internal need am I meeting with my limit or abundance of expression?
- 🗣 I can now allow myself to freely be me. I am now safe and loved.
- ⊙ Imagine removing any obstructions from your mind, heart, and gut. See these areas as free to express.

F

Facade: (see Hiding)

- 🔹 Black Pepper, Kumquat, Vetiver, Deep Blue®, Helichrysum, Cinnamon, Juniper Berry

Failing:

- 🔹 Bergamot, Roman Chamomile, Cumin, Green Mandarin
- ⬇ What does success look like? Would it serve to change my definition of success?
- 🗣 I now reject belittling thoughts about myself. I now accept success.
- ⊙ Imagine drawing every needful thing toward yourself, all things being provided abundantly. Imagine harmonizing with your higher purposes.

Faith:

- 🔹 Sandalwood, Immortelle, Hope®, Cheer®, Turmeric, Laurel Leaf
- ⬇ What experience is causing me to question my belief? What will it take for me to see the truth of things?

- ◀ᵈ I reject all falsehood. I now believe in myself and the abundant good surrounding me. It is now safe for me to listen to my inner voice of truth.
- ⊙ See light dispel darkness from around your body. Invite this light to dispel all false thinking and lift your mind to clarity.

Family Traditions: (see *Generational Healing*)

Father, Connection to:
- ♦ Frankincense, Amāvī®
- ⇩ Do I feel let down by my father? What does my inner child crave?
- ◀ᵈ I am now valued, protected, and loved.
- ⊙ See your notions of fatherhood. Imagine discarding what is not serving, while honoring all the good.

Fatigued, Mentally:
- ♦ Lemon, Rosemary, Dill, PastTense®, Lemon Myrtle
- ⇩ What am I unsettled about? What will it take for me to come to peace with this situation?
- ◀ᵈ I can now release unnecessary details and trust that the solution is working itself out.
- ⊙ See the chaos around your brain settle into organized compartments that are accessible if needed. Imagine allowing your brain to breathe.

Fatigued, Physically: (see *Exhausted*)

Fearful:
- ♦ Brave®, Juniper Berry, Cassia, Cinnamon, Birch, Cypress, Lavender, Myrrh, Spikenard, Peppermint, Deep Blue®, Cumin, Peace®, Green Mandarin, Yarrow | Pom, Turmeric, Black Spruce, Adaptiv®, Davana
- ⇩ What is the root of my fear? What will it take for me to process this fear?
- ◀ᵈ I now release fear. I now trust that I am safe and provided for today and in my future.
- ⊙ See a light dispel darkness around your body. Invite this light to dispel all false thinking, and lift your mind to higher truth about the self and the future.

♦ Oils   ⇩ Look Deeper   ◀ᵈ Declare   ⊙ Visualize

Fearless: (see *Courageous*)

Firm: (see *Resolute*)
- ♦ Clove, Birch

Flexible:
- ♦ Cypress, AromaTouch®, Wild Orange, Birch, Oregano
- ⇩ What am I afraid of? What do I fear losing?
- ◁ᴱ I can now flow with life. All things now work together for my good.
- ⊙ See yourself release your grasp on the cords which constrict your movement.

Flighty: (see *Ungrounded*)

Focused:
- ♦ Lemon, Rosemary, Spearmint, Thinker®, ᵈᵒᵀᴱᴿᴿᴬ Balance®, InTune®, Lemon Myrtle
- ⇩ What am I avoiding? What is causing me to feel overwhelmed?
- ◁ᴱ I am now present and laser focused. I am now granted vision beyond my own.
- ⊙ See gray mist lift from around your head. See a ray of light fill your mind and pour through your eyes.

Food, Preoccupation with: (see *Dieting, Obsession with*)

Foolish:
- ♦ Cassia, Spearmint, Blue Tansy
- ⇩ What am I choosing to avoid? What will it take for me to process the discomfort I feel?
- ◁ᴱ I can and will now listen to my inner voice and follow its lead.
- ⊙ See gray mist lift from around your head. See a ray of light fill your mind and vision.

Forgetful: (see *Distracted*)
- ♦ Lemon, Peppermint

Forgiven:
- ♦ Copaiba, Siberian Fir, Geranium, Red Mandarin
- ⇩ Am I carrying hurt which is not serving me? What is holding me back from extending forgiveness to myself or others?
- ◁ᴱ I can now ask for forgiveness. I now allow myself to be forgiven and free.

EMOTIONS

- ⊙ See cords unwind and release from around your heart and body. Imagine the lungs expanding with newfound freedom.

Forgiving:
- ♦ Geranium, Thyme, Forgive®, Siberian Fir, Holiday Peace®, Citronella
- ⇩ Am I carrying hurt which is not serving me? What is holding me back from extending forgiveness to myself or others?
- ◀» I am now open to forgive myself and others. I now release hurt and allow full healing into my life.
- ⊙ See cords unwind and release from around your heart and body. Imagine your hands and heart letting go of hurt.

Frantic: (see Hurried)

Friendless: (see Limiting Beliefs)
- ♦ Marjoram, Cedarwood, Birch

Frustrated:
- ♦ Geranium, Cardamom, Neroli, Roman Chamomile
- ⇩ What am I trying to control? What is this trigger teaching me?
- ◀» I can now embrace life and easily flow with its twist and turns, for it is leading me to higher paths and purposes.
- ⊙ Imagine your hands letting go of control. See your body flow with, and navigate around, anything you may encounter on your life's path.

Fulfilled:
- ♦ Roman Chamomile, Tangerine, Jasmine, Neroli, Star Anise
- ⇩ Am I connected to my Higher Power? What am I craving?
- ◀» Everything I need now draws to me in freely.
- ⊙ See your open arms being filled with love and healing. See all that you need flowing toward you.

G

Generational Healing:
- ♦ Black Spruce, Cedarwood, Douglas Fir, Petitgrain, Holiday Peace®, Red Mandarin, TerraShield®

♦ Oils   ⇩ Look Deeper   ◀» Declare   ⊙ Visualize

⇩ Am I ready to be free of generational grievances and change my future course? What will it take to stop trying to fix others?

🔊 I am now free of the past, and I can now move forward with purpose.

⊙ See your connection to past generations. Imagine discarding the connections that are not serving, while keeping all of the beauty.

Generational Issues: (see *Generational Healing*)

◆ Petitgrain, Birch, Douglas Fir, Jasmine, DDR Prime®, Holiday Peace®, Amāvī®, Black Spruce, Forgive®, Citronella

Generous:

◆ Wild Orange, Magnolia

⇩ Is it possible the more I give, the more I receive? Do I have limiting beliefs that are self-sabotaging?

🔊 I now choose to be generous with my time, money, and judgments. I make the world a better place.

⊙ Imagine healing hands placed over your heart to hold and heal it. Feel pure love renewing your heart and extending out to others.

Gentle:

◆ Geranium, Ylang Ylang, Whisper®

⇩ What experience do I need to process through? Am I feeling physically or emotionally vulnerable?

🔊 I can now trust that I am held in safety and protection.

⊙ See a soothing cloth placed around your body to calm and quiet your mind, heart, and gut.

Giving Up: (see *Defeated*)

◆ Hope®, Helichrysum, Deep Blue®

Gladness: (see *Cheerful*)

◆ Tangerine, Sunny Citrus, Wild Orange, Cheer®, Ylang Ylang

Good Enough: (see *Worthy*)

Grace:

◆ Arborvitae, Rose, Frankincense, Wintergreen, Immortelle, Manuka

⇩ What will it take to realize that I always have access to divine help and strength? What has caused me to believe I should do everything through my own strength?

🔊 I can now allow grace to carry me.

⊙ See yourself step into the light of grace. Listen to your breath. Imagine laying down anything that is no longer serving you.

Grateful:

♦ Spikenard, Wild Orange, Helichrysum, PastTense®, Douglas Fir, Lime, Manuka, Magnolia, Beautiful, Harvest Spice®

⇩ Do I recognize the good in my life? Do struggles make me feel important?

🔊 I can now recognize and prize the good in my life.

⊙ See the good things in life magnified and enhanced in your mind's eye. Invite more good to enter the space.

Greedy: (see Abundant)

♦ Wild Orange, Spikenard

Grieving:

♦ Breathe®, Deep Blue®, Geranium, Lime, Ylang Ylang, AromaTouch®, Manuka, Console®, Siberian Fir

⇩ What did I lose? What will it take to process that loss and move forward?

🔊 I am now finding new hope each day. I can now allow grace to carry me.

⊙ See a weight lifting off the chest, allowing your lungs to expand and receive an abundance of pure oxygen and light.

Grounded:

♦ Balance®, Birch, Steady®, Patchouli, Vetiver, Arborvitae, Myrrh, InTune®, Hinoki, Amāvī®, Magnolia, Black Spruce, Niaouli

⇩ Am I living in the past or the future? What will it take to be connected to the here and now? What am I protecting myself from?

🔊 I am now grounded in the present.

⊙ See yourself as a kite, anchored to a steady point which allows you to safely soar.

Guarded:

♦ ClaryCalm®, Jasmine

⇩ What experience do I need to process through? Am I feeling physically or emotionally vulnerable? (see Defensive)

♦ Oils   ⇩ Look Deeper   🔊 Declare   ⊙ Visualize

Guilty:
- ♦ Copaiba, Bergamot, Lemon, Peppermint, Citrus Bloom®
- ⇩ What do I feel responsible for? Is this accurate? What will it take for me to move forward from guilt?
- ◄ᴵ⁾ I am now open to learn the truth about this situation. I am now filled with virtuous love for myself and others.
- ⊙ See yourself disposing of a bag of dark muck. See strong wind clearing out the dust particles in your body and filling it with virtue and kindness.

H

Happy:
- ♦ Citrus Bliss®, Elevation, Cheer®, Green Mandarin, Sunny Citrus, Lime, Lemon, Peppermint, Ylang Ylang, Spikenard
- ⇩ What did I lose (hit to the ego, loss of material possession, relationship)? What will it take for me to trust that the Universe is supporting me?
- ◄ᴵ⁾ I am now capable of moving forward in joy. I now claim a happy heart.
- ⊙ See darkness retreat from your body. Imagine bright sunshine flowing over the front of your body, into the crown of your head, and along the spine.

Harassed: (see *Attacked*)

Hardened:
- ♦ Rose, Geranium, Ylang Ylang, Tangerine, Jasmine
- ⇩ What didn't go as planned? What will it take for me to stop protecting myself from the future? What will it take for me to allow my future to be different from my past.
- ◄ᴵ⁾ I now validate past hurt and am now ready for a newness of life.
- ⊙ See yourself removing a protective layer from around your heart. Imagine nurturing surrounding your heart.

Hardhearted: (see *Hardened*)
- ♦ Rose, Geranium, Thyme

Harsh: (see *Hardened*)
- ♦ Marjoram, Geranium, Cardamom

Hateful:

🜄 Thyme, Purify, Cardamom

⇩ How was I hurt? How does holding on to this hurt continue to harm me?

🔊 I can now offer and receive forgiveness daily. I am now filled with charity toward all people.

⊙ Imagine yourself letting go of the person or situation that hurt you. As you do, imagine a rush of water flowing through your body, filling you with love, light, and forgiveness.

Haunted: (see *Reassured*)

🜄 Frankincense, On Guard®, Melissa, Yarrow | Pom

Healing:

🜄 Helichrysum, Geranium, Eucalyptus, Breathe®, Jasmine, Rose, Ylang Ylang, Deep Blue®, Manuka, Hope®, Console®, Turmeric, Magnolia, Beautiful

⇩ What caused my hurt? What gift has this brought me?

🔊 I now surrender to healing.

⊙ Imagine yourself filled with light and healing. See support flowing into the body wherever it is needed.

Healthy: (see *Whole*)

🜄 DDR Prime®, Eucalyptus, Basil

Heard:

🜄 Lavender, Spearmint

⇩ Who am I seeking to please or receive validation from? Do I trust and love myself?

🔊 I am now cherished, valued, and respected.

⊙ See yourself filled up with divine love. You might imagine this as a color or feeling flowing into or surrounding your body. Feel your muscles release tension and your breathing open.

🜄 Oils   ⇩ Look Deeper   🔊 Declare   ⊙ Visualize

Heartbroken:
- 🜄 Geranium, Rose
- ⇩ Why did this experience cause so much hurt? How can this be applied to my growth?
- 🔊 I can now let go of sorrow. I am now open to love.
- ⊙ Imagine healing hands placed over your heart to hold and heal it. Feel pure love renewing your body.

Heartless: (see *Connected, Emotionally*)
- 🜄 Geranium, Rose

Heavyhearted: (see *Heartbroken*)
- 🜄 Lime, Elevation, Geranium, Tangerine, Peppermint, Rose, Cheer®, Green Mandarin

Helpless:
- 🜄 Clove, Ginger, On Guard®, Cheer®, Yarrow | Pom
- ⇩ What decisions need to be made so I can move forward? What will it take for me to get the help I need?
- 🔊 I can now accept the help I need. I am open to seeing the solutions ready for me.
- ⊙ See a force move through you from behind to propel you forward and upward on your journey. Imagine being lifted over any obstacles in your way.

Hereditary Issues: (see *Generational Issues*)

Hesitant: (see *Indecisive*)

Hiding:
- 🜄 Cassia, Black Pepper, Lavender, Spearmint, Grapefruit, Juniper Berry, Siberian Fir, Kumquat, Anchor, Tamer®, Laurel Leaf
- ⇩ Who or what am I hiding from? What causes me to feel like I can't reveal that part of myself? Why do I feel vulnerable?
- 🔊 I am now safe. I now resonate with truth. I am now open to healing.
- ⊙ Imagine yourself removing a protective covering from around your body. See comforting light fill up any areas in the mind, heart, or body that feel vulnerable.

Hoarding: (see *Obsessed*)
- Lemongrass, Purify, Zendocrine®, Wild Orange

Holding Back: (see *Apprehensive*)
- Cassia, Lavender, Spearmint, Jasmine

Holding On to Past: (see *Stuck*)
- Thyme, Lemongrass, Purify, Zendocrine®, Wintergreen, Siberian Fir, Holiday Peace®

Honest:
- Black Pepper, Geranium, Lavender, Lime, Kumquat, Siberian Fir
- ⇩ Who or what am I hiding from? What causes me to feel like I can't reveal a part of myself? Why do I feel vulnerable?
- ◀᫟ I am now safe. I now resonate with truth. I am now open to healing.
- ☉ Imagine comforting light fill up any areas in the mind, heart or body that feel vulnerable.

Hopeful:
- Melissa, Lime, Bergamot, Helichrysum, Immortelle, Motivate®, Hope®, Cheer®, Green Mandarin, Turmeric
- ⇩ What is causing me to feel stuck? What do I believe is outside my control?
- ◀᫟ I am now filled with gratitude and hope for my future.
- ☉ Imagine yourself looking through special glasses that give you true perspective about the path you are on. See gratitude flood your heart.

Hopeless: (see *Hopeful*)
- Hope®, Melissa, Clary Sage, Bergamot, Helichrysum, Lime, Cheer®, Green Mandarin, Turmeric

Humble: (see *Arrogant*)
- Oregano, Sandalwood

- Oils   ⇩ Look Deeper   ◀᫟ Declare   ☉ Visualize

Humiliated:

♦ Cassia

⇩ What caused me to feel humiliated? What will it take to forgive myself?

🔊 It is now safe for me to learn and make mistakes. I now accept myself.

⊙ Imagine surrendering the box of humiliation that was once inside your body. Allow love to fill its place.

Humor, Sense of: (see *Joyful*)

♦ Wild Orange, Elevation, Ylang Ylang, Sunny Citrus

Hurried: (see *Hurried*)

♦ AromaTouch®, PastTense®, Serenity®, Hinoki, Holiday Peace®, Magnolia

Hurtful:

♦ Forgive®, Rose, Thyme

⇩ What caused my hurt? What will it take for me to process the hurt into healing?

🔊 I now surrender my hurt and open to healing.

⊙ Imagine yourself filled with light and healing.

Hypocritical: (see *Hiding*)

♦ Kumquat, Clary Sage, Frankincense, Black Pepper

Hysterical: (see *Panicked*)

I

Illness, Attached to:

♦ Eucalyptus, Patchouli

⇩ (see *Self-punishing*)

Imbalanced: (see *Balanced*)

♦ Serenity®, Citrus Bliss®, PastTense®, Hinoki, Align, Magnolia, Align, Celery Seed, Calmer®

Immature:

♦ Geranium, Fennel

⇩ Is there something in me that needs to express or be heard so I can move forward? What am I running away from?

◀ᴹ I am now safe and willing to listen to my inner child. I am now patient with myself.

⊙ Imagine allowing your inner child to express. See your inner child and current self make peace with each other.

Immobilized: (see *Stuck*)

Impatient:
🌢 Balance®, Thyme, Neroli
⇩ What am I nervous about? Do I trust that things work out for me?
◀ᴹ I now release all nervousness; I am now filled with peace and perspective.
⊙ Imagine nervous energy vacuumed away from your body. See clear water washing over your body and bringing peace.

Impoverished: (see *Abundant*)
🌢 Wild Orange, Spikenard

Imprisoned: (see *Trapped*)

Impulsive: (see *Agitated*)
🌢 Sandalwood, Vetiver, Jasmine

Inadequate: (see *Self-acceptance*)
🌢 Bergamot, Slim & Sassy®, Pink Pepper, Beautiful

Inauthentic: (see *Authentic*)
🌢 Kumquat, Black Pepper, Steady®

*Incapable: (*see *Capable*)
🌢 Bergamot, Lemon, Peppermint, Steady®, Rosemary, Cassia, Rescuer

Inconsiderate: (see *Kind*)
🌢 Cinnamon, Forgive®, Spikenard, Cumin

Inconsistent: (see *Empowered*)
🌢 Balance®, Coriander

🌢 Oils ⇩ Look Deeper ◀ᴹ Declare ⊙ Visualize

Indecisive: (see *Decisive*)
- Lemon, Peppermint, Lemon Myrtle

Independent: (see *Empowered*)
- On Guard®, Clove

Indifferent: (see *Apathetic*)

Inferior:
- Bergamot, Pink Pepper
- What is causing me to feel that I am less than I should be? Who or what has taught me this? What will it take for me to let go of the shoulds in my life that do not serve?
- I am now whole and complete, perfectly and divinely designed.
- Imagine yourself dismissing the thoughts that are not serving. See love and light transform your perspective. Listen to your breath.

Inflexible: (see *Rigid*)

Initiative: (see *Courageous*)
- Blue Tansy

Innocent: (see *Childlike*)
- Ylang Ylang, Geranium, Jasmine, Red Mandarin, Green Mandarin

Insecure:
- Cassia, Bergamot, Cinnamon, Lemon, Citrus Bliss®, Lavender, Pink Pepper
- What will it take for me to be enough regardless of the approval of others? Do I trust my inner voice?
- I now believe in my ability to move forward. I am now safe, secure, and abounding in grace.
- Imagine yourself wrapped in peace. See your feet anchored to a comforting pathway; imagine confidence flowing from the path up your body. See your feet intuitively move forward.

Insensitive: (see *Defensive*)
- Cumin, Oregano

Insignificant: (see *Worthy*)
- Roman Chamomile

Inspired:
- ⬥ Passion®, Roman Chamomile, Lemon, Rosemary, Elevation, Blue Tansy, Arise, Green Mandarin, Turmeric
- ⇩ What will it take for me to connect to the inspiration waiting for me? What life experiences have caused me to limit myself?
- ◀» I am now open to infinite possibilities. Solutions are now waiting for me.
- ⊙ See light pouring from the sacral chakra/reproductive area of your body. Visualize a gift being handed to you that contains ideas beyond your own. See your mind expanding to hold more.

Instability: (see *Stable*)
- ⬥ Balance®, Anchor

Integrated: (see *Adjusting*)
- ⬥ Dill, Arise, Holiday Peace®, Magnolia, Tamer®, Tulsi

Integrity: (see *Authentic*)
- ⬥ Coriander, Black Pepper, Melissa, On Guard®, Kumquat, Pink Pepper, Align, Amāvī®

Intimate: (see *Sexuality, Healthy*)

Intimidated: (see *Boundaries*)
- ⬥ Clove, TerraShield®, Ginger, Yarrow | Pom

Intolerant: (see *Defensive*)
- ⬥ Geranium, Rose, Thyme, Cardamom, Forgive®

Introverted: (see *Safe*)
- ⬥ Marjoram, Cedarwood

Intuitive:
- ⬥ Clary Sage, Litsea, Blue Tansy, Arise
- ⇩ What will it take for me to trust my inner voice? What am I protecting it from?
- ◀» I am now allowed to trust myself.
- ⊙ Imagine unlocking any restraints that are holding back your intuition. See your mind, heart, and gut connect and work together in harmony to support your intuitive flow.

| ⬥ Oils | ⇩ Look Deeper | ◀» Declare | ⊙ Visualize |

Invigorated: (see *Energized*)
- Peppermint, Lemon, Citrus Bliss®

Invulnerable: (see *Protected*)
- ClaryCalm®, Marjoram

Irrational: (see *Rational*)
- Cardamom, Juniper Berry, Deep Blue®

Irresponsible: (see *Responsible*)
- Fennel, Ginger, Balance®

Irritated:
- Forgive®, Whisper®, Citronella
- ⇩ What trigger caused my agitation? What does this trigger reveal about my subconscious beliefs? Am I ready to be honest with myself about my limiting beliefs?
- ◀ᴵ I now release the pain of the past. I am now open to healing and wholeness.
- ⊙ Imagine looking for holes inside your mind, heart, or body. Choose a nurturing color to fill up and soothe these holes.

Isolated:
- Marjoram, Cedarwood, Myrrh, Magnolia, Harvest Spice
- ⇩ What am I protecting myself from? What will it take for me to process the harm I experienced in the past?
- ◀ᴵ I now accept the truth that I am safe and loved. It is now safe for me to connect with others.
- ⊙ Imagine yourself removing protective gear from your body. Imagine restorative light and love surrounding you.

J

Jaded:
- Red Mandarin, Spikenard
- ⇩ What didn't turn out as I expected? Do I have more to express before I move on from that experience? What will it take for me to release the past and be open to receive new outcomes?
- ◀ᴵ I now validate pain from my past. I am now ready and willing to be open to new outcomes.

⊙ Imagine jaded memories removed from your mind and body. Imagine the remaining space being washed clean.

Jealous:
◆ Cinnamon, Wild Orange, Sandalwood, Oregano
⇩ Is it possible that I can be successful while another is successful? Do I feel loved and accepted?
◀ᴼ I am now filled with charity. I now choose to see the best in others.
⊙ Imagine removing a blindfold from your eyes. See charity and gratitude flowing through your body toward all others on your path.

Joyful:
◆ Lemon, Lime, Wild Orange, Tangerine, Peppermint, Ylang Ylang, Citrus Bliss®, Elevation, Melissa, Red Mandarin, Holiday Joy™, Cheer®, Sunny Citrus, Green Mandarin, Arise, Citrus Bloom®
⇩ Do I have permission from myself to feel joy? Am I grieving over a loss? Do I feel loved and accepted?
◀ᴼ I am now open to joy. I can now move forward with vigor and optimism.
⊙ Imagine removing all things attached to or around your body that are blocking joy. See a ball of light fill the vacated area and flow throughout your body.

Joyless: (see *Joyful*)
◆ Elevation, Lemon, Ylang Ylang, Tangerine, Melissa, Red Mandarin, Passion®, Cheer®, Wild Orange, Green Mandarin, Arise

Judged: (see *Betrayed*)
◆ Birch, Clove, Ginger, Cassia

Judgmental: (see *Acceptance*)
◆ Geranium, Rose, Black Pepper, Forgive®, Pink Pepper, Citronella

Justifying: (see *Responsible*)
◆ Magnolia

◆ Oils   ⇩ Look Deeper   ◀ᴼ Declare   ⊙ Visualize

EMOTIONS

K

Kind:

- Geranium, Whisper®, Neroli, Pink Pepper
- Am I kind to myself or others? How was I hurt? How does holding on to this hurt continue to harm me?
- I choose to offer and receive forgiveness daily. I am now filled with charity toward everyone around me.
- See yourself offer a laurel wreath to the person or situation that hurt you. As you do, see healing waters flow through your body, filling you with love, light, and forgiveness.

Know-it-all: (see *Competitive*)

- Oregano, Wintergreen, Sandalwood

L

Learning issues: (see *Learning* in Body Guide)

- Lemon, Rosemary, DigestZen®

Left Out: (see *Isolated*)

Lethargic: (see *Connected, Physically*)

- Lemongrass, Citrus Bliss®, Blue Tansy

Liberated:

- Zendocrine®, Purify, Lavender, Melissa, Eucalyptus, Cilantro, Green Mandarin, Adaptiv®
- Am I forcing a connection that is not serving me? Can I trust that I will be directed to relationships that will serve me?
- I am now permitted and free to release all distorted thinking and limiting beliefs. I can now listen to my inner voice of truth.
- See your body open to reveal all the goodness inside. Imagine oxygen flowing in to strengthen and multiply that goodness until you are filled with royal light.

Lighthearted: (see *Joyful*)

Limiting Beliefs:

- Zendocrine®, Lemongrass, Bergamot, Vetiver, Litsea, Green Mandarin

💧 What life experiences have caused me to limit myself? Is it possible that these limiting beliefs are not founded in truth?

🔊 I now release false notions and limiting expectations for myself and others. I am now open to infinite possibilities.

⊙ See yourself release any cords preventing you from moving forward. Imagine divine wind carrying you forward to fulfill your life's mission and purpose.

Lonely: (see *Isolated*)

💧 Marjoram, Cedarwood, Frankincense, Myrrh

Longing:

💧 Immortelle, Rose, Magnolia, Helichrysum, Breathe®, Console®, Siberian Fir, Frankincense, Myrrh,

💧 Am I connected to my higher purposes? What am I craving?

🔊 Everything I need now draws to me freely.

⊙ Imagine a covering of love and reassurance placed around your heart and body; it may appear as brilliant light or soft, comforting fabric.

Loss of Will to Live:

💧 Hope®, Citrus Bliss®, Melissa, Frankincense, Lime, Elevation

💧 What is causing me to give up my power to act? Have I asked for help to release what is binding me?

🔊 I am now open to movement and flow. There is now purpose for me.

⊙ See rushing water wash all heaviness from around your body. Consider physical movement to support.

Loss: (see *Grieving*)

💧 Geranium, Ylang Ylang, Console®, Siberian Fir

Lost: (see *Purposeless*)

💧 Oils   💧 Look Deeper   🔊 Declare   ⊙ Visualize

Loved:
- ♦ Frankincense, Rose, Breathe®, Myrrh, Bergamot, Marjoram, Manuka, Beautiful, Niaouli
- ⇩ Am I connected to my higher purposes? What am I craving?
- ◀ I can now accept that I am infinitely loved.
- ⊙ Imagine looking for holes inside your mind, heart, or body. Choose a nurturing color to fill these holes with love.

Loving:
- ♦ Rose, Geranium, Marjoram, Forgive®, Pink Pepper, Align, Bergamot Mint
- ⇩ What experience caused hurt? Is this blocking my ability to love? Am I ready to release this pain?
- ◀ I can now let go of sorrow and open myself to love.
- ⊙ See kind hands placed over your heart to hold and heal it. Imagine a renewing of your heart.

Loyal:
- ♦ Petitgrain, Jasmine, Neroli
- ⇩ Am I safe to trust others? Do I trust myself? Am I loyal to my highest goals and purposes?
- ◀ I now choose to be loyal to my divine purposes. I am now supported in every moment.
- ⊙ Imagine a covering of love and reassurance placed around your heart and body; it may appear as brilliant light or soft, comforting fabric.

Lustful:
- ♦ Cinnamon, Jasmine
- ⇩ What is empty in me? What am I trying to numb? What am I avoiding confronting?
- ◀ I am now balanced and free. I now determine my destiny.
- ⊙ See yourself peeling off and then tossing aside those habits which act as chains that bind. Consider inviting divine help to weaken the chains and fill the soul with true purpose and meaning.

M

Mad: (see *Angry*)

Manifesting:
- ◆ Litsea, Green Mandarin
- ⬇ Am I afraid of my own brilliance? What has taught me to fear success?
- ◀ᵚ I no longer fear my own brilliance. I can now manifest miracles.
- ⊙ Identify faulty notions in your mind and heart. Remove these ideas to make room for dreams and goals to flourish.

Manipulated: (see *Violated*)
- ◆ Clove, On Guard®, Yarrow | Pom

Manipulative: (see *Jealous*)
- ◆ Cinnamon, Kumquat, Pink Pepper, Cumin, Cilantro, Cypress

Masculine, Overly: (see *Insecure*)
- ◆ Whisper®, ClaryCalm®, Amāvī®

Materialistic: (see *Emptiness*)
- ◆ Sandalwood, Oregano, Cilantro, Zendocrine®

Mean:
- ◆ Geranium, Ylang Ylang, Neroli
- ⬇ Who or what has hurt me? Am I defending myself by acting in a mean way? What will it take for me to process the hurt I feel?
- ◀ᵚ I am now trading hurt for healing.
- ⊙ Imagine peeling hurt off of your body. See healing balm soothe your body, mind, and heart.

Melancholy: (see *Sad*)

Menopause, Dread of: (see *Fear*)
- ◆ ClaryCalm®, Grapefruit, Jasmine

Menstruation, Dread of: (see *Fear*)
- ◆ ClaryCalm®, Grapefruit, Jasmine

Misaligned: (see *Aligned*)

◆ Oils   ⬇ Look Deeper   ◀ᵚ Declare   ⊙ Visualize

Misunderstood:
- Spearmint, Lavender, Cedarwood, Birch, Copaiba, Manuka, Whisper®, ClaryCalm®, Litsea
- Am I forcing a connection that is not serving me? What will it take to create relationships that will serve me?
- I am now free and willing to release all distorted thinking and limiting beliefs.
- See a blanket of comfort lovingly placed around your body. Imagine its presence allows trust and calm to absorb into the soul.

Moderation: (see *Balanced*)
- Patchouli

Mother, Connection to:
- Myrrh, Whisper®, ClaryCalm®
- Do I feel let down by my mother? What does the inner child crave?
- I am now open to understanding the magnificence of motherhood.
- See your notions of motherhood. Imagine discarding what is not serving, while honoring all of the good.

Motivated: (see *Empowered*)
- Citrus Bliss,® Black Pepper, Dill, Motivate®, Blue Tansy, Green Mandarin

N

Narrow-minded: (see *Closed-minded*)

Negative Habits: (see *Self-sabotage*)
- Zendocrine®, DDR Prime®, Grapefruit, Black Pepper

Neglected: (see *Nurtured*)
- Myrrh, Cedarwood, Marjoram

Nervous:
- Basil, Wild Orange, PastTense®, Spearmint
- What future event worries me? What am I afraid I will lose?
- I am now accepting serenity and clarity. I can now trust in the rightness of my life.
- Imagine peaceful light flow around and through you like a river.

Nightmares: (see *Sleep* in Body Guide)
- Juniper Berry, Black Spruce, Clary Sage

Nonattachment:
- Oregano, Sandalwood, Cilantro, Wintergreen, Lemongrass, Spikenard, Cumin
- Who or what am I protecting myself from? Is it possible my nervous system is stuck in a survival response?
- I am now perfectly supported in every moment. I am now open to experiencing safe connection.
- See a blanket of peace placed around your body. Imagine its presence allows trust and calm to absorb into the soul.

Nourished: (see *Nurtured*)
- Grapefruit, Myrrh, DigestZen®

Numb: (see *Traumatized*)
- Fennel, Magnolia

Nurtured:
- Myrrh, Rose, Frankincense, Geranium, Ylang Ylang, ClaryCalm®, Magnolia, Niaouli
- What will it take for me to see myself as worthy or receiving the time, attention, and love I need? What will it take for me to assign greater value to my own needs, wants, and ideas?
- I am now cherished, valued, and worthy of love, time, and attention.
- See kind hands placed over your heart to hold and heal it. Imagine a renewing of your heart.

O

Objective: (see *Open-minded*)
- Cardamom, Thyme, Pink Pepper

- Oils   Look Deeper   Declare   Visualize

Obsessed:

- Cilantro, Grapefruit, Patchouli, Zendocrine®, Frankincense, Elevation, Peppermint, Vetiver, Arborvitae, Adaptiv®, Forgive®, Jasmine, Basil
- What is the root of my worry? What do I feel I need to control?
- I am now clearing my mind to receive new knowledge and thought. I am now an agent who acts, not one who is acted upon.
- Imagine brushing everything off of you that is not yours to hold. See yourself letting go of control on all levels.

Obsessive-compulsive: (see *Obsessed*)

- Cilantro, Cypress, Adaptiv®, Peace®, Bergamot, Sandalwood, Black Pepper, Purify, Jasmine

Offended: (see *Unforgiving*)

Open-minded:

- Clary Sage, Wild Orange, AromaTouch®, Rosemary, Thyme, Green Mandarin, Align
- What life experience has taught me that it is unsafe to try new things? Am I open to ideas outside of my box? What one step can I take today to move toward achieving my goals?
- I can now release all fear. I am now open to doing things differently. I now have unseen support at every turn.
- See your eyes illuminate things unseen, allowing your mind to be filled with new ideas.

Opinionated: (see *Competitive*)

- Oregano

Oppressed: (see *Violated*)

- Clove, On Guard®, White Fir, Turmeric

Optimistic:

- Melissa, Citrus Bliss®, Tangerine, Bergamot, Peppermint, Elevation, Sunny Citrus, Siberian Fir, Green Mandarin, Arise, Turmeric, Citrus Bloom®
- Why did life events not go my way? Is it possible this new way opens to better things than what I had planned?
- I can now believe and receive abundance.
- See a bright beam of light aimed right at your heart, bringing new

energy and uplift to your body, mind, and spirit.

Out of Control:
- ♦ Balance®, Ginger, Steady®, Jasmine
- ⇩ What am I trying to control? What am I afraid of? Do I have a need to be perfect?
- ◀» I no longer need to expect perfection. I can now accept things the way they are.
- ☉ See chaos removed from around your body. Feel a flow of ordered energy and light enter your body from the crown of your head, and move down through the bottom of your feet.

Out of Integrity: (see *Aligned*)
- ♦ Align, Coriander

Over-analyzing: (see *Anxious*)
- ♦ Wild Orange, Ylang Ylang, Sandalwood, Basil, Adaptiv®

Over-stimulated: (see *Nervous System* in Body Guide*)
- ♦ DigestZen®, Balance®, Thinker®, Dill, Hinoki, Lemon Myrtle, Magnolia

Overthinking: (see *Overanalyzing*)

Overwhelmed:
- ♦ Basil, AromaTouch®, Rescuer, PastTense®, DigestZen®, Tangerine, Melissa, Red Mandarin, Serenity®, Yarrow | Pom, Tamer®, Island Mint®
- ⇩ What am I trying to control? Do I trust that help outside myself is readily available?
- ◀» I am now perfectly supported in every moment. All things now work together for my good.
- ☉ See white light flooding into your heart and supporting the spine and low back.

Overworked: (see *Workaholic*)

♦ Oils   ⇩ Look Deeper   ◀» Declare   ☉ Visualize

P

Pain, Emotional:

♦ Helichrysum, Hope®, Manuka, Deep Blue®, Geranium, Peppermint, Console®, HD Clear®

⇩ What false beliefs hold me captive?

◄⁑ I now surrender all sadness and open myself to healing.

⊙ See darkness retreat from your body. Imagine bright sunshine flow over the front of your body, into the crown of your head, and along the spine.

Pain, Resisting: (see *Pain, Emotional*)

♦ Deep Blue®, Helichrysum, Vetiver

Panicked:

♦ Balance®, Deep Blue®, Adaptiv®

⇩ What triggered these feelings of fear? What is causing my lack of trust?

◄⁑ Fear is a liar. I am now perfectly supported.

⊙ See a blanket of comfort lovingly placed around your body. Imagine its presence allows trust and calm to absorb into the soul.

Passionate:

♦ Jasmine, Fennel, Passion®, Davana

⇩ What emotions are weighing me down? What do I feel responsible for? What will it take to listen to my inner voice?

◄⁑ I now know my life has purpose and meaning. I am now ready to fulfill my higher purposes.

⊙ Imagine a spark ignite in your heart, filling your body with energy. See intention flow from you to accomplish your desires and purposes.

Passive-aggressive:

♦ Kumquat, Cilantro

⇩ What will it take for me to ask for what I really need and want? What will it take for me to listen and heed my inner voice?

◄⁑ I now choose to be honest about my needs and no longer repress my emotions.

⊙ See a blanket of love and comfort placed around the body. Allow calm to absorb into the soul.

Patient:
- ♦ Balance®, Thyme, Neroli, Forgive®, Serenity®, Magnolia, Niaouli
- ⇩ What am I nervous about? Do I trust that things work out for me?
- ◀)) I now release all nervousness; I am now filled with peace and perspective.
- ⊙ Imagine nervous energy vacuumed away from your body. See cleansing water washing over your body and bringing peace.

Peaceful:
- ♦ Peace®, Serenity®, Roman Chamomile, Calmer®, Patchouli, Copaiba, Siberian Fir, Hinoki, Holiday Peace®
- ⇩ What will it take for me to live in integrity with my values? What needs to change so that I can experience greater peace?
- ◀)) I can now trust that all things will work together for my good.
- ⊙ See a blanket of love and comfort placed around the body. Allow calm to absorb into the soul.

Peer Pressure: (see *Controlled*)

Perceptive: (see *Intuitive*)
- ♦ Magnolia, Clary Sage, Immortelle, Melissa

Perfectionistic: (see *Distrusting*)
- ♦ Cypress, Serenity®, Sunny Citrus, Amāvī®

Persecuted: (see *Attacked*)

Persevering: (see *Resolute*)
- ♦ Helichrysum, Balance®, Hope®

Perspective: (see *Clarity, Mental*)
- ♦ Siberian Fir, Red Mandarin, Frankincense, Clary Sage, Holiday Peace®, Turmeric, Magnolia

Pessimistic: (see *Apprehensive*)
- ♦ Spikenard, Wild Orange, Peppermint, Tangerine, Forgive®, Sunny Citrus, Arise

♦ Oils   ⇩ Look Deeper   ◀)) Declare   ⊙ Visualize

Pioneering:
- ♦ Petitgrain, Roman Chamomile, Litsea
- ⇩ What will it take to trust my inner voice and move forward in faith? Am I open to ideas outside of my box? What one step can I take today to move toward achieving my goals?
- ◁⁾ I can now release any fear of being the first. I have unseen support at every turn.
- ⊙ Imagine yourself surrendering to the encouraging wind propelling your body in a forward motion.

Playful: (see *Carefree*)
- ♦ Ylang Ylang, Wild Orange, Tangerine, Elevation, Passion®, Sunny Citrus

Poor, financially: (see *Impoverished*)

Possessive: (see *Controlling*)
- ♦ Sandalwood, Oregano, Wintergreen

Powerless:
- ♦ Clove, Ginger, Jasmine, Manuka, Tea Tree, Star Anise
- ⇩ What caused me to relinquish my power to act? What benefits do I receive when I remain a victim? What is *my* dream?
- ◁⁾ I now claim my power to act. I am powerful and ready to choose for myself.
- ⊙ Imagine a spark ignite in your heart, filling your body with energy. See intention flow from you to accomplish your desires and purposes.

Present: (see *Grounded*)
- ♦ InTune®, Ginger, Lemon, Patchouli, Siberian Fir, Vetiver, Balance®, Holiday Peace®, Anchor, Magnolia, Harvest Spice

Pretense: (see *Superficial*)

Prideful: (see *Arrogant*)
- ♦ Oregano, Sandalwood, Wintergreen, Black Pepper

Proactive: (see *Empowered*)
- ♦ Clove, Fennel

Procrastinating:

💧 Blue Tansy, InTune®

⬇ What do I need to process through so I am free to move forward? Do I have a good balance of work and rest? What am I afraid of?

🗨 I can now move forward with confidence and ease. All things now come together for my good.

⊙ Imagine yourself being propelled forward by rushing waters that carry you effortlessly to where you need to go.

Protected:

💧 On Guard®, Clove, TerraShield®, Frankincense, Stronger®, Juniper Berry, Yarrow | Pom, Lemon, Eucalyptus, Niaouli

⬇ Are my boundaries strong? What will it take for me to honor my space (mental, physical, emotional) and allow others to stay in their own space? Do I have a healthy understanding of what is and is not okay for me?

🗨 I no longer need to allow unwelcome influences into my space. I can now honor my boundaries by refusing them.

⊙ Imagine yourself in a protective bubble that completely covers the space around your body. See yourself fill the space with positive colors and emotions.

Purifying:

💧 Purify, Lemongrass, Jasmine, Zendocrine®, Lemon Myrtle

⬇ What is ready to be dismissed from my life (thoughts, relationships, activities)?

🗨 I am now ready and willing to receive what is fresh and clean.

⊙ Take a deep breath, allowing your lungs to inhale freshness and exhale what is no longer serving.

Purposeful:

💧 Roman Chamomile, Ginger, Blue Tansy, Copaiba, Litsea

⬇ What is causing me to give up my power to act? What will it take to connect with my inner voice of truth?

🗨 I am now open to movement and flow. There is great purpose for me.

⊙ See rushing water washing all heaviness from around your body. Imagine wind lifting and propelling your body in an upward, forward motion.

💧 Oils   ⬇ Look Deeper   🗨 Declare   ⊙ Visualize

Purposeless
- ◆ Roman Chamomile, Frankincense
- ⇩ What is missing in my life? Who can help me find the direction I am seeking? Am I in need of physical or emotional direction?
- ◀» I know who I am and I am now filled with confidence and faith in my future.
- ☉ See yourself standing strong and immovable, grounded on a golden pathway of abundance, with the light of truth flowing through the crown of your head and filling your body.

Q

Quarrelsome: (see *Argumentative*)

Quick-tempered: (see *Angry*)
- ◆ Geranium, Cardamom

Quitting:
- ◆ Helichrysum, Hope®
- ⇩ How did life events not go my way? Is it possible that this new way opens to better things than what I had planned?
- ◀» I will not be conquered.
- ☉ See a bright beam of light enter your heart, bringing new energy and flow to your body, mind, and spirit.

R

Raging: (see *Angry*)
- ◆ Cardamom, Thyme, Purify, Turmeric

Rational:
- ◆ Lemon, Cardamom, Dill, Niaouli
- ⇩ What do I feel the need to escape from? Is there something I don't want to see about my life? What comforts me about living in a fantasy world?
- ◀» I now easily navigate living in the real world. I am now connected and safe.
- ☉ Imagine yourself as a tree. See roots anchored in the earth, reassuring and connecting your mind and body to the present moment.

Reassured:

♦ Peace®, Yarrow | Pom, Helichrysum, Calmer®, Black Spruce, Star Anise, Anchor, Steady®, Siberian Fir, Adaptiv®

⇩ What experience do I need to process through? Is it ready to be released?

◀๑ I can now accept that life events whether good or ill, uncover the best in me and lead to my greatest happiness.

⊙ Imagine a soothing cloth calming and quieting your mind, heart, and gut.

Rebelling: (see *Defensive*)

♦ Fennel, Bergamot, Copaiba, Forgive®, Coriander, Spikenard, Amāvī®

Rebirth: (see *Transforming*)

♦ DDR Prime®, Helichrysum, Hope®

Reclusive: (see *Isolated*)

♦ Marjoram, Cedarwood

Refreshed: (see *Renewed*)

Regretful: (see *Grieving*)

♦ Copaiba, Siberian Fir

Rejection:

♦ Lavender, Cinnamon, Lime, Clove, Marjoram, ClaryCalm®, Litsea

⇩ Am I the one rejecting or am I being rejected? Have I felt rejected by another? What might be limiting that person from giving the love I seek?

◀๑ I can now accept that I am loved and valued. I am now ready to love myself.

⊙ See yourself surrounded and held by loving, white light.

EMOTIONS

Relationships:

🌢 Neroli, Tea Tree, On Guard®, Oregano, Jasmine, Geranium, Marjoram, Cedarwood, Holiday Peace®, Amāvī®

⬇ What will it take for me to enjoy healthy relationships in my life? Do I love and value myself?

🗣 I am now open to beautiful relationships that fill my life with joy.

⊙ See a blanket of peace placed around your body. Imagine its presence allows trust and calm to absorb into the soul.

Relaxed: (see *Calm*)

🌢 PastTense, Adaptiv®, Serenity®, Lavender, Roman Chamomile, AromaTouch®, Arborvitae, Elevation, Hinoki, Island Mint

Relieved: (see *Liberated*)

🌢 Helichrysum, PastTense®, Peppermint

Reluctant:

🌢 Brave®, Fennel, Blue Tansy, Ginger, Tamer®, Motivate®, Lavender, Cypress

⬇ What is causing me to fear making a choice and moving forward? When did this start?

🗣 I can now claim my power to choose.

⊙ Imagine the weight of fog lifted from around your head, allowing fresh sunlight and oxygen to illuminate your mind with ideas.

Renewed:

🌢 Basil, Peppermint, Red Mandarin, Star Anise, Green Mandarin, Magnolia, Bergamot Mint

⬇ What is ready to be dismissed from my life (thoughts, relationships, activities)?

🗣 I am now refreshed and ready for life.

⊙ Take a deep breath, allowing your lungs to inhale freshness and exhale what is no longer serving.

Repressed: (see *Violated*)

🌢 Lavender, Vetiver, Black Pepper, Jasmine, Kumquat, Ylang Ylang, Star Anise

Resentful:

🌢 Geranium, Thyme, Forgive®, Neroli

EMOTIONS

How was I hurt by another? What struggle within that person may have caused them to spread their hurt to me?

I can now forgive and forget. My heart now expands in love and gratitude.

Imagine your heart held in perfect love. As it is held, see it empty of sludge to expand and receive healing.

Resigned: (see *Despairing*)

Resilient: (see *Renewed*)
- Tea Tree, Helichrysum, Lime, Deep Blue®, Neroli, Copaiba, Turmeric

Resisting: (see *Defensive*)
- Vetiver, Deep Blue®, Spikenard, DigestZen®, Fennel, Whisper®, Amāvī®

Resolute:
- Birch, Spearmint, Black Spruce, Brave®
- What causes me to doubt my decisions? What first caused me to doubt my ability to choose for myself?
- I am now allowed to be decisive. Direction now flows easily.
- Imagine yourself with a continuous stream of light flowing through your mind, heart, and gut. See yourself perfectly illuminated with the knowledge needed to move forward.

Respectful:
- Cardamom, Douglas Fir, Tea Tree, Cumin, Magnolia, Brave®, Beautiful
- Do I respect myself? Do I live consist with my understanding of right and wrong?
- I now choose to surround myself with that which uplifts and inspires.
- See darkness lifted off the front of your body. Imagine reassuring currents of love flowing over your body, bringing forgiveness and new life.

- Oils   ⇩ Look Deeper   ◀)) Declare   ⊙ Visualize

Responsible:
- ♦ Ginger, Fennel, Balance®, Eucalyptus, Blue Tansy, Turmeric
- ⇩ What caused me to relinquish my power to act? What benefits do I receive when I remain a victim? Do I need to clarify my role in order to move forward?
- ◄꙱ I can now claim my power to act. I am powerful and ready to choose for myself.
- ⊙ Imagine confidence absorbing into your feet. See your feet instinctively move forward.

Restless: (see *Agitated*)
- ♦ Serenity®, Console®, Neroli, Lavender

Restored: (see *Renewed*)
- ♦ Turmeric, Celery Seed

Revitalized: (see *Energized*)

Rigid:
- ♦ Cypress, Oregano, Wild Orange, Tangerine, AromaTouch®, Hinoki
- ⇩ What will it take for me to recognize there are many right ways to do something? Am I defending against a real or perceived threat? Am I ready to consider other options that might serve me or those around me?
- ◄꙱ I can now release all fear. I am now open to doing things differently. I now have unseen support at every turn.
- ⊙ See your eyes illuminate things unseen, allowing your mind to be filled with new ideas.

Rushed: (see *Hurried*)

S

Sacrificing: (see *Victim Mentality*)
- ♦ Sandalwood, Wintergreen, Arborvitae

Sad:
- ♦ Breathe®, Ylang Ylang, Geranium, Peppermint, AromaTouch®, Elevation, Siberian Fir
- ⇩ What did I lose (hit to the ego, loss of material possession, relationship)? What may I gain from this experience?
- ◄꙱ I now choose to move forward in joy. I now claim a happy heart.

⊙ See darkness retreat from your body. Imagine bright sunshine flowing over the front of your body, into the crown of your head, and along the spine.

Safe:

♦ Myrrh, Frankincense, Lavender, Breathe®, On Guard®, Tea Tree, Manuka, Holiday Joy™, TerraShield®, Yarrow | Pom, Adaptiv®, Niaouli

⇩ Am I feeling physically or emotionally vulnerable? Do I trust something larger than myself for protection and safety?

◄ᵑ I am now held in safety and protection. I am now constantly inspired with direction for my life.

⊙ Imagine a continuous stream of light flowing through your mind, heart, and gut. See yourself illuminated with the knowledge needed to move forward.

Scarcity: (see *Abundant*)

♦ Wild Orange, Spikenard, Cumin

Scattered:

♦ Vetiver, Balance®, Spearmint, InTune®, Yarrow | Pom, Holiday Peace®

⇩ What is necessary for me to process, and what can I let go? Do the details of life clamor for my attention?

◄ᵑ I can now trust my body to filter and put in order what is necessary for success. I now release all messages not serving me.

⊙ Imagine all low-vibrating matter fall away from your body and mind. Breathe in order and peace.

Secure: (see *Protected*)

Self-acceptance:

♦ Bergamot, Grapefruit, Slim & Sassy®, Lemon, Jasmine, Patchouli, Hope®, HD Clear®, Pink Pepper, Align, Adaptiv®, Bergamot Mint

⇩ What will it take to approve of myself? What will it take for me to assign honor and value to myself?

◄ᵑ I now choose to value and honor myself and invite others to do the same.

⊙ Imagine identifying and dismissing false notions about yourself. Take a moment to honor who you truly are.

♦ Oils   ⇩ Look Deeper   ◄ᵑ Declare   ⊙ Visualize

Self-assured: (see *Confident*)

Self-aware: (see *Intuitive*)
- 🜄 Juniper Berry, HD Clear®, Copaiba, Kumquat, Pink Pepper, Arise

Self-betrayal:
- 🜄 Coriander, Kumquat, Black Pepper, Litsea
- ⬇ Have I rejected myself? What will it take for me to heal my relationship with myself?
- 🗩 I can now trust that I am embraced and valued.
- ⊙ Imagine a covering of love and reassurance placed around your heart and body.

Self-centered: (see *Generous*)
- 🜄 Cumin, Spikenard, Oregano

Self-comparison:
- 🜄 Pink Pepper, Bergamot, Thyme
- ⬇ Who am I trying to please? What is causing me to fear moving forward?
- 🗩 I can now trust my internal compass. I now choose to move forward in confidence and faith.
- ⊙ See yourself dismiss the conflicting voices on either side. See light pouring over your head and face.

Self-control:
- 🜄 Cardamom, Thyme, Oregano, Slim & Sassy®, Ginger, Deep Blue®
- ⬇ What causes me to feel like I am not in control? Has someone or something taught me that I have no power?
- 🗩 I am now ready to determine my own destiny. My choices and actions now lead me where I want to go.
- ⊙ See chaos removed from around your body. Feel a flow of ordered energy and light enter your body from the crown of your head, and move down through the bottom of your feet.

Self-critical:
- 🜄 Slim & Sassy®, Bergamot, Litsea, Pink Pepper, Beautiful, Adaptiv®
- ⬇ What am I punishing myself for? What do I need to process through so that I can forgive and let go of negative thinking? Am I trusting false thoughts?

◀))) I am now ready and willing to surrender belittling self-talk. I can now allow myself to be cherished and held dear.
⊙ See yourself lay down all weapons of self harm, receiving grace in return.

Self-deception: (see *Hiding*)
◆ Black Pepper, Pink Pepper

Self-doubt: (see *Self-esteem*)

Self-esteem:
◆ Bergamot, Slim & Sassy®, Cassia, Jasmine, Litsea, Pink Pepper, Green Mandarin, Beautiful, Laurel Leaf
⇩ Do I have negative self-talk? How is this self-talk a distortion of what is really true? Am I willing to stop letting distorted thoughts or my perception of what others think of me dictate my reality?
◀))) I am now ready and willing to surrender belittling self-talk. I am now open to learning the truth about my brilliance.
⊙ Imagine that dark colors or distorted shapes are swept from your mind, heart, and gut. Replace these with shapes and colors that lift and inspire.

Self-expression: (see *Hiding*)
◆ Lavender, Citrus Bliss®, Spearmint, Jasmine, Star Anise

Self-judgment: (see *Self-critical*)
◆ Bergamot, Slim & Sassy®, Lemon, HD Clear®, Pink Pepper

Self-punishing: (see *Self-critical*)
◆ Bergamot, Slim & Sassy®, Jasmine

Self-sabotage:
◆ Slim & Sassy®, Zendocrine®, Blue Tansy, Marjoram
⇩ Am I afraid of my own brilliance? What has taught me to fear success?
◀))) I can now release fearing my own brilliance. I reject all belittling self-talk.
⊙ Identify and dismiss faulty notions in your mind and heart. Invite positive beliefs to provide fresh support.

◆ Oils   ⇩ Look Deeper   ◀))) Declare   ⊙ Visualize

Self-worth: (see *Self-esteem*)

♦ Pink Pepper, Bergamot, Rosemary, Grapefruit, Manuka

Self, True to: (see *Authentic*)

♦ Align, Coriander, Lavender, Birch, Black Pepper, Clove, On Guard®, Kumquat, Pink Pepper, Star Anise

Self, Weak Sense of: (see *Self-esteem*)

♦ Bergamot, Vetiver, Ginger, Balance®, Fennel, Jasmine

Selfish:

♦ Spikenard, Magnolia, Rose

⇩ What will it take for my needs to be met? Are my expectations of my needs balanced or making up for a lack I feel in other areas of my life?

◁》 I can now trust that there is more than enough. I can now trust I will receive everything I need.

⊙ Take a deep breath. See yourself receive all needed love, nurturing, and care.

Sensitive, Overly:

♦ TerraShield®, On Guard®, Clove, Ginger, Holiday Joy™

⇩ What is necessary for me to process, and what can I let go? Do multiple messages clamor for my attention?

◁》 I can now trust my body to filter and put in order what is necessary for success. I now reject all messages not serving me.

⊙ Imagine all low-vibrating matter fall away from your body and mind. Feel your strength increase.

Separated: (see *Connected, Emotionally*)

♦ Myrrh, Frankincense, Cedarwood, Manuka, Magnolia

Serious, overly:

♦ Tangerine, Citrus Bliss®, Elevation, Wild Orange, Passion®, Sunny Citrus, Lemon Myrtle, Yarrow | Pom, Green Mandarin

⇩ What emotions are weighing me down? What do I feel responsible for?

◁》 I can now surrender all my cares. I am now free to release responsibilities that are not mine.

⊙ Imagine water wash out the heavy darkness from your body.

Feel lightheartedness enter your heart and mind.

Sexual Fixation: (see *Sexuality, Imbalanced*)

Sexual Identity: (see *Sexual Health* in Body Guide)
- Cinnamon, Jasmine

Sexuality, Healthy: (see *Sexual Health* in Body Guide)
- Cinnamon, Whisper®, Patchouli, Jasmine, Neroli, Amāvī®, Davana

Sexuality, Imbalanced: (see *Sexual Health* in Body Guide)
- Cinnamon, Whisper®, Jasmine, Neroli, Amāvī®, Davana

Sexuality, Repressed: (see *Sexuality, Imbalanced*)

Shameful:
- Copaiba, Bergamot, Frankincense, Fennel, Cassia, Jasmine, Hope®
- What is my first experience with shame? What false belief in me fosters these feelings? Am I ready to release this pattern in my life and receive feelings of worthiness?
- I am now filled with love and gratitude for my life experiences. My Higher Power teaches me of my great worth.
- Imagine all sludge draining out of your body through the lower back. See love and light entering through the crown of your head, filling the entire body.

Shock:
- Basil, Peppermint, Wintergreen
- What experience do I need to process through? Is this ready to be released?
- I can now trust beauty and goodness to flow into my life. I am now filled with gratitude and new hope for the future.
- See a soothing cloth calm and quiet your mind, heart, and gut.

- Oils   ⇩ Look Deeper   ⊲⁾ Declare   ⊙ Visualize

Shy:

- ⬥ Cassia, Spearmint, Cinnamon, Ginger
- ⬇ What do I wish to hide from others? Who or what has taught me my words, ideas, or life is less than others? Is my fear of making a mistake keeping me from creating rewarding relationships?
- ◀ I am now ready and willing to release fear of others' judgments. I now honor me!
- ⊙ See any shyness exit your body. Consider if it is covering something else up.

Sincere: (see *Honest*)

- ⬥ Kumquat, Black Pepper

Sleep, Disrupted: (see *Sleep* in Body Guide)

- ⬥ Juniper Berry, AromaTouch®

Soothed: (see *Comforted*)

Speaking, Fear of: (see *Fearful*)

- ⬥ Spearmint, Lavender

Spiritual:

- ⬥ Frankincense, Arborvitae, Manuka, Sandalwood, Rose, Roman Chamomile, Immortelle
- ⬇ What is allowing darkness to enter in my life (such as negative thought patterns or practices)? What do I need to change in my life to be more aligned with my Higher Power?
- ◀ I now cast off all negative or lower vibrational energies and fill myself with light and truth.
- ⊙ Imagine a dark mist or cloud around you being dispelled by light and faith.

Spiritual Blindness: (see *Spiritual*)

- ⬥ Immortelle, Clary Sage, Lemongrass, Frankincense, Yarrow | Pom

Spontaneous: (see *Carefree*)

- ⬥ Wild Orange, Citrus Bliss®, Tangerine, Passion® ᵈᵒᵀᴱᴿᴿᴬ, Sunny Citrus

Stable:

- ⬥ Balance® ᵈᵒᵀᴱᴿᴿᴬ, Patchouli, ClaryCalm®, Elevation, Hinoki, Anchor, Amāvī®, Turmeric, Magnolia, Black Spruce, Chamomile, Immortelle
- ⬇ What future event worries me? What am I afraid I will lose?

💧 I am now accepting serenity and clarity. I can now trust in the rightness of my life.

⊙ Imagine a steady, calming light flowing around and through you like a river.

Stagnant: (see *Stuck*)

Stern: (see *Serious, Overly*)

Still:

💧 Sandalwood, Arborvitae, Immortelle, Peace®, Holiday Peace®, Align

⬇ What will it take for me to be at peace with my conscience or inner self? What will it take for me to give myself permission to take the time to be still?

💧 I am now accepting serenity and clarity. I can now trust in the rightness of my life.

⊙ Imagine a steady, calming light flowing around and through you like a river.

Strengthened:

💧 Birch, On Guard®, Stronger®, Wintergreen, Balance®, Deep Blue®, Basil, Peppermint, Star Anise, Yarrow | Pom, Amāvī®, Turmeric

⬇ What is causing drag in my life? Have I taken the time to nurture myself? Am I aligned with my mission and purpose in life?

💧 I now accept my strength and capabilities to move forward with passion and purpose.

⊙ Imagine confidence absorbing into your feet and enlivening your body. See your feet instinctively carry you forward.

Stressed:

💧 AromaTouch®, Serenity®, Ylang Ylang, Adaptiv®, PastTense®, Basil, Vetiver, Red Mandarin, Holiday Joy™, Sunny Citrus, Hinoki, Amāvī®

⬇ Am I carrying burdens that are not my own? What will it take to live in the present moment and leave the future to itself? What will it take to have realistic expectations for myself?

💧 I am now adopting the belief that all things work together for my good.

⊙ Imagine peace flowing down through your body. See light encircle your body. Listen to your breath.

💧 Oils   ⬇ Look Deeper   💧 Declare   ⊙ Visualize

Stubborn:

♦ Wintergreen, Oregano

⇩ What am I trying to control? What do I fear losing?

◁» I can now flow with life. All things now work together for my good.

⊙ See yourself slide chains off your wrists and feet. Imagine flying forward to newfound freedom.

Stuck:

♦ Cypress, Lemongrass, Thyme, Birch, Fennel, Cilantro, Ginger, Purify, Zendocrine®, DDR Prime®, Motivate®, Sunny Citrus, Neroli, Green Mandarin, Citrus Bloom®

⇩ What do I need to process through? What do I need to give up in order to experience transformation?

◁» I can now move forward with confidence and ease. All things now come together for my good.

⊙ Imagine ropes unwind and release from around your heart and body. Imagine cutting through any lies and distortion being held by the mind or heart.

Suffering: Manuka, Cheer®, Whisper®

Superficial: (see *Hiding*)

♦ Black Pepper, Oregano, Coriander, Kumquat

Supported:

♦ Birch, Cedarwood, Arborvitae, Roman Chamomile, Breathe®, Manuka, Yarrow | Pom, Anchor

⇩ What will it take for me to trust the process of life? What am I trying to control?

◁» I am now perfectly supported in every moment.

⊙ Imagine allowing yourself to be led forward by grace and strength beyond your own.

Suppressing: (see *Hiding*)

♦ HD Clear®, Copaiba, Geranium, Star Anise, Davana

Surrender:

♦ Wintergreen, Spikenard, Sandalwood, Arborvitae

⇩ What am I trying to compensate for? What is unfulfilled in me?

◁» I am now filled with acceptance for what I cannot change, courage

to change what I can, and wisdom to know the difference.
- ⊙ Imagine brushing everything off of you that is not yours to hold. See yourself letting go of control on all levels.

Sympathetic: (see *Understanding*)
- ♦ Neroli, Geranium, Marjoram, Forgive®

T

Teachable:
- ♦ Wintergreen, Oregano, Rosemary, Magnolia, Niaouli
- ⇩ Am I safe to admit that I do not know everything? Is it possible there are undiscovered ideas and concepts that may serve me?
- ◁⋙ I am now open to new ideas and patterns. I can now trust that good flows to me.
- ⊙ Imagine a flow of light and knowledge washing false beliefs out of the mind and heart. See the mind and heart comforted in love and acceptance.

Tenderhearted: (see *Gentle*)
- ♦ Geranium, Ylang Ylang, Rose

Tense:
- ♦ AromaTouch®, PastTense®, Cypress, Lavender, ClaryCalm®, Serenity®, Hinoki
- ⇩ What am I protecting myself from? What will it take for me to process the harm I experienced in the past?)
- ◁⋙ I am now perfectly supported in every moment. I am now open to trusting that I am safe to be me.
- ⊙ See yourself remove protective gear from your body. Imagine restorative light and love surrounding you.

Terrified:
- ♦ Juniper Berry, Yarrow | Pom
- ⇩ What voices am I listening to? Do they uplift and inspire me to higher purposes?
- ◁⋙ I now choose faith. I now have unseen support in every moment.
- ⊙ Imagine comfort surrounding and calming the body and mind. Feel your breathing steady to a supportive rhythm.

| ♦ Oils | ⇩ Look Deeper | ◁⋙ Declare | ⊙ Visualize |

Thankful: (see *Grateful*)

Timid: (see *Shy*)

Tired: (see *Exhausted*)

Tolerant:
- Thyme, Geranium, Deep Blue®, Cardamom, Forgive®, Neroli, Pink Pepper
- ⇩ Am I clear on what is safe for me to accept? Am I protecting myself from something?
- ◁⍦ I now have permission to honor my boundaries.
- ⊙ See yourself align with your inner compass and the highest good for you. Feel your shoulders release tension.

Toxic: (see *Purifying*)
- Lemongrass, Tea Tree, Purify, Zendocrine®, Cilantro, Lime, Thyme, DDR Prime®, Lemon Myrtle, Celery Seed

Transforming:
- Helichrysum, Deep Blue®, Elevation, Immortelle, DDR Prime®, Citrus Bloom
- ⇩ Am I satisfied with the status quo? What do I need to give up in order to experience transformation?
- ◁⍦ I can now listen to the quiet voice of truth within me. I am now transforming step by step.
- ⊙ See yourself shed old, unhelpful patterns and embrace new gifts and abilities.

Transitioning: (see *Adjusting*)

Trapped: Petitgrain, Lavender, Thyme, Purify, Cilantro, Black Pepper, Zendocrine®, Eucalyptus, Jasmine, Elevation, Green Mandarin

Traumatized:
- Hope®, Geranium, Clove, Helichrysum, Ylang Ylang, Jasmine, Console®, Yarrow | Pom
- ⇩ What caused shock to my system? Have I allowed myself enough time to process and release? Am I patient with myself?
- ◁⍦ I can now trust beauty and goodness to flow into my life. I am now filled with gratitude and new hope for the future.

- ⊙ See yourself being held and comforted by perfect love. Listen to your breath and trust your healthy biological impulses.

Trusting:
- ♦ Geranium, Marjoram, Myrrh, Rosemary, Jasmine, Cypress, Arborvitae, Breathe®, Immortelle, Rose, Manuka, Turmeric, Align, Adaptiv®, Davani, Niaouli
- ⇩ What am I protecting myself from? How has my ego been harmed?
- ◀ᵈ I now choose faith. I now have unseen support in every moment.
- ⊙ See yourself lay down the defenses you have been holding onto and step into grace.

U

Unashamed: (see *Shameful*)
- ♦ Cassia, Copaiba

Unattractive: (see *Self-acceptance*)
- ♦ Grapefruit, Slim & Sassy®

Uncertain:
- ♦ Anchor, Clary Sage, Copaiba
- ⇩ Have I been unpleasantly surprised by life in the past? What will it take for me to feel assured?
- ◀ᵈ I can now move forward in faith. I am now perfectly supported.
- ⊙ See yourself as a tree with roots anchored in rich, nourishing soil, receiving everything needed to be safely sustained.

Unclean: (see *Purifying*)
- ♦ Frankincense, Detoxification, Purification, Lemongrass

Unclear:
- ♦ Yarrow | Pom
- ⇩ What am I worrying about which causes me to feel unsafe or conflicted? Have I been unpleasantly surprised by life in the past?
- ◀ᵈ I can now anchor to truth. I am now resolved and safe in this present moment.
- ⊙ Imagine ropes unwinding and releasing from around your heart and body. See a sword of truth cutting through any lies and distortion.

♦ Oils   ⇩ Look Deeper   ◀ᵈ Declare   ⊙ Visualize

Unconscious: (see *Unconscious* in Body Guide)

🌢 Petitgrain, Marjoram, TerraShield®

Understanding:

🌢 Thyme, Cardamom, Forgive®

⇩ Who am I seeking to please or receive validation from? Do I trust and love myself enough to extend that love to others?

🔊 I am now cherished, valued, and respected.

⊙ See yourself filled up with divine love. You might imagine this as a color or feeling flowing into or surrounding your body. Feel your muscles release tension and your breathing open.

Unfocused: (see *Focused*)

🌢 Lemon, Thinker®, Peppermint, InTune®, Lemon Myrtle

Unforgiving:

🌢 Thyme, Geranium, Forgive®, Rose

⇩ Am I carrying hurt which is not serving me? What is holding me back from extending forgiveness to myself or others? Am I ready to be free of generational grievances and change my future course?

🔊 I am now open to forgiving myself and others. I now release hurt and allow full healing into my life.

⊙ See water wash out the heavy darkness from your body and imagine sunshine renewing every cell.

Unfulfilled: (see *Fulfilled*)

🌢 Roman Chamomile, Jasmine, Neroli, Litsea

Ungrateful: (see *Grateful*)

🌢 Spikenard, Wild Orange, Helichrysum, PastTense®, Douglas Fir, Lime

Ungrounded: (see *Grounded*)

🌢 Balance®, Patchouli, Vetiver, Hinoki, Amāvī®

Unhealthy: (see *Whole*)

🌢 Celery Seed, Eucalyptus

Unheard: (see *Heard*)

🌢 Lavender, Spearmint

Unified: (see *Aligned*)

🌢 Magnolia, Cedarwood, Rose, Marjoram

Unkind: (see *Mean*)

Unloved: (see *Loved*)
- Bergamot, Breathe®, Lavender, Rose, Jasmine, Hope®

Unloving: (see *Loving*)
- Geranium, Rose, Thyme

Unmotivated: (see *Motivated*)
- Motivate®, Citrus Bliss®, Blue Tansy, Litsea, Black Pepper, Dill

Unnurtured: (see *Nurtured*)
- Myrrh

Unprotected: (see *Protected*)
- On Guard®, TerraShield®, Frankincense, Manuka, Yarrow | Pom, Lemon Eucalyptus

Unsafe: (see *Safe*)
- Myrrh, On Guard®, Jasmine, Frankincense, Tea Tree, Manuka, Peace®, Yarrow | Pom, Turmeric

Unseen: (see *Hiding*)

Unsettled: (see *Stable*)
- Roman Chamomile, Console, Anchor, Rescuer

Unstable: (see *Stable*)
- Anchor, Black Spruce, Steady®, Turmeric

Unsupported:
- Birch, Cedarwood, Arborvitae
- What is interfering with me trusting the process of life? What will it take for me to receive the support I need?
- I can now accept that I am perfectly supported in every moment.
- Imagine support flowing down the spine. See it fill the body with strength and nurturing.

Unsympathetic: (see *Heard*)

- Oils   ⇩ Look Deeper   ◀ Declare   ⊙ Visualize

- Neroli, Geranium, Magnolia

Unteachable:
- Rosemary, Oregano

Unworthy:
- Copaiba, Cassia, Hope®, Slim & Sassy®, Laurel Leaf
- Are the voices I am listening to from a trustworthy source? What is clouding my perspective of myself? What does my Higher Power tell me about my worthiness? Are there things I need to change?
- I can now accept that I have intrinsic worth and value. I can now harmonize my life with my highest good.
- Imagine surrendering all unworthiness. See your mind, heart, and gut be filled with perfect love.

Unyielding: (see *Stubborn*)

Upheaval: (see *Transitioning*)
- Anchor, Steady®, Balance®, Adaptiv®, Black Spruce

Upheld: (see *Supported*)
- Manuka, Yarrow | Pom, Adaptiv®

Uplifted: (see *Energized*)
- Cheer®, Melissa, Tangerine, Star Anise, Arise™, Bergamot Mint

V

Valued: (see *Worthy*)

Victim Mentality:
- Clove, Ginger, Spikenard, Jasmine, On Guard®, Copaiba
- What will it take for me to stop blaming other people and situations for my unhappiness? Am I ready to see the truth about myself and my power to act? Do I have unresolved hurt?
- I can now accept full responsibility for my own happiness. I no longer need to blame others.
- See yourself being released from a heavy burden. Feel the freedom of exploring the world around you with a fresh perspective.

EMOTIONS

Violated:

♦ On Guard®, Ginger, Clove, Jasmine

⇩ Are my boundaries strong? What will it take for me to honor my space (mental, physical, emotional) and allow others to stay in their own space? Do I have a healthy understanding of what is and is not okay for me?

◂� I no longer need to allow unwelcome influences into my space. I can now honor my boundaries by refusing them.

⊙ Imagine yourself in a protective bubble that completely covers your body, mind, and spirit. Imagine nurturing and healing light flowing into that protected space.

Violent: (see *Angry*)

♦ Peace®, Frankincense, Cardamom

Vulnerable:

♦ ClaryCalm®, On Guard®, TerraShield®, Jasmine, Niaouli

⇩ Am I feeling physically or emotionally vulnerable? Do I trust something larger than myself for protection and safety?

◂ᴹ I am now held in safety and protection. I now believe that I am constantly inspired with direction for my life.

⊙ See a blanket of peace placed around your body. Imagine its presence allows trust and calm to absorb into the soul.

W

Weak-willed:

♦ Petitgrain, Birch, Tea Tree, Ginger, Clove, Wintergreen

⇩ What caused me to relinquish my power to act? What benefits do I receive when I remain a victimized? What is *my* dream?

◂ᴹ I can now claim my power to act. I am powerful and ready to choose for myself.

⊙ See water wash out the heavy darkness from your body and imagine sunshine renewing every cell.

Weary: (see *Exhausted*)

Well: (see *Immune System* in Body Guide)

♦ Eucalyptus, Patchouli, Fennel, Celery Seed

♦ Oils   ⇩ Look Deeper   ◂ᴹ Declare   ⊙ Visualize

Whole:
- ♦ Helichrysum, Manuka, Rose, Copaiba, Console®, Star Anise, Arise™, Magnolia
- ⬇ What is causing me to feel that I am less than I should be? Who or what has taught me this?
- 🔊 I now dismiss any negativity in or around me. I am now ready to heal.
- ⊙ Imagine dismissing any negativity in the mind, heart and body. See yourself being filled with love and light.

Willful: (see *Defensive*)
- ♦ Oregano, Wintergreen, Arborvitae

Wisdom:
- ♦ Douglas Fir, Frankincense, Petitgrain, Siberian Fir, Holiday Peace®
- ⬇ Am I ready to apply the lessons life has taught me? Am I in integrity with my inner voice? What is blocking my good judgment?
- 🔊 I now apply the lessons of my life experience to the present moment. I can now rely on my good judgment.
- ⊙ Visualize light flowing from the crown of your head and out your eyes. Imagine this light flowing over your brain, heart, and gut.

Withdrawn: (see *Isolated*)

Workaholic:
- ♦ Wild Orange, Ylang Ylang, Tangerine, Basil, PastTense®, Cedarwood
- ⬇ Am I running away from something that I do not want to confront? What will it take for me to recognize what is off-balance in my life? Am I using my work to escape pain?
- 🔊 I am now ready and willing to see the truth.
- ⊙ Imagine brushing off your hands of everything that is not yours to hold. See yourself trusting that all essentials are provided for.

Worried:
- ♦ Calmer®, Wild Orange, Tangerine, Sandalwood, Cilantro, Peace®, AromaTouch®, Elevation, Adaptiv®

💧 Do I doubt myself? Am I relying solely on my own strength? What will it take to trust I have the support I need?

🔊 I am now perfectly supported in every moment. I can now move forward in confidence and strength.

⊙ See a light turned on in your mind, illuminating what does not belong. See yourself make room to receive greater light and perspective.

Worthless:

💧 Cassia, Bergamot, Slim & Sassy®

💧 Is this a feeling that will help me progress or turn to my Higher Power? Is it possible this feeling does not originate from a source of truth?

🔊 I can now reject falsehood. I am now cherished, valued, and worthy of infinite love.

⊙ Imagine yourself held in loving arms. See what value you truly hold. Imagine your heart open to receive all the love that is yours.

Worthy:

💧 Bergamot, Slim & Sassy®, HD Clear®, Copaiba, Beautiful®

💧 Am I trusting in false thoughts about myself? What is clouding my perspective of myself? What am I to change?

🔊 I was born with intrinsic worth and value. I now reject belittling thoughts about myself.

⊙ See your heart, mind, and gut surrender any feelings of unworthiness and be filled with love. Open your arms to receive all that is yours.

Wounded: (see Hurtful)

💧 Helichrysum, Manuka, Jasmine, Deep Blue®, Hope® doTERRA

💧 Oils 💧 Look Deeper 🔊 Declare ⊙ Visualize

NEGATIVE EMOTIONS
& POSITIVE PROPERTIES

ESSENTIAL OIL	NEGATIVE EMOTIONS	POSITIVE PROPERTIES
SINGLE OILS		
ARBORVITAE	Overexerting Struggling Distant from God	Grace-filled Trusting Peaceful Surrender
BASIL	Fatigued Depleted Dependent	Energized Renewed Rested
BERGAMOT	Self-judgment Insecure Unloved	Self-acceptance Optimistic Confident
BERGAMOT MINT	Disappointed Exhausted Rejecting self	Uplifted Refreshed Self-acceptance
BIRCH	Unsupported Weak-willed Alienated	Supported Resolute Connected
BLACK PEPPER	Superficial Hiding Self-deception	Honest Authentic Courageous
BLACK SPRUCE	Unstable Depleted Fearful	Stable Resolute Grounded
BLUE TANSY	Procrastinating Resisting Apathetic	Inspired Initiative Motivated
CARDAMOM	Angry Aggressive Disrespectful	Objective Self-control Respectful
CASSIA	Fear of rejection Shy Timid	Courageous Unashamed Valued

ESSENTIAL OIL	NEGATIVE EMOTIONS	POSITIVE PROPERTIES
CEDARWOOD	Separate Aloof Lonely	Connected Belonging Social
CELERY SEED	Toxic Sluggish Stagnant	Restored Cleansed Well
CILANTRO	Controlling Worried Trapped	Unattached Cleansing Liberated
CINNAMON	Fear of rejection Sexual repression Pretense Jealousy	Attractive Healthy sexuality Intimate Accepting
CITRONELLA	Irritated Judgmental Invaded	Averting Discerning Forgiving
CLARY SAGE	Confused Limited Blocked	Clarity Intuitive Imaginative
CLOVE	Controlled Self-betrayal Codependent Poor boundaries	Empowered Clear boundaries Protected
COPAIBA	Guilty Self-loathing Regretful	Forgiven Worthy Redefined
CORIANDER	Controlled Self-betrayal Disloyal	Integrity Inner guidance True to self
CUMIN	Unbridled ambition Self-centered Scarcity	Balanced ambition Respectful Abundant thinking
CYPRESS	Rigid Perfectionistic Controlling	Trusting Flowing Adaptable

EMOTIONS

ESSENTIAL OIL	NEGATIVE EMOTIONS	POSITIVE PROPERTIES
DAVANA	Inhibited Passionless Suppressed	Creative Passionate Flowing
DILL	Bored Disinterested Overstimulated	Engaged Motivated Integrated
DOUGLAS FIR	Repeating mistakes from the past Generational patterns Negative traditions	Wisdom Respectful Generational healing Healthy connections
EUCALYPTUS	Afflicted Depleted Despondent Defeated	Well Responsible Liberated
FENNEL	Irresponsible Loss of appetite Body neglect	Responsible Satiated In tune
FRANKINCENSE	Darkness Deceived Spiritually disconnected Abandoned	Wisdom Discerning Spiritually connected
GERANIUM	Distrusting Grieving Broken-hearted	Trusting Loving Tolerant Open
GINGER	Victim mentality Blaming Powerless	Empowered Capable Responsible
GRAPEFRUIT	Body judgment Disrespecting body Obsession with food or dieting	Body acceptance Respect for body Meeting physical needs
GREEN MANDARIN	Fearful Burdened Trapped Limited	Fearless Excited Hopeful Limitless potential
HELICHRYSUM	Traumatized Wounded Hopeless	Whole Courageous Hopeful

ESSENTIAL OIL	NEGATIVE EMOTIONS	POSITIVE PROPERTIES
HINOKI	Disharmonious Energetically blocked Hurried	Harmonious Balanced Calm
JASMINE	Resistant Sexual fixation Sexual issues	Intimate Pure Healthy sexuality
JUNIPER BERRY	Terrified Fearful Nightmares	Protected Courageous Dreaming
KUMQUAT	Inauthentic Passive aggressive Hiding	Authentic Honest Sincere
LAUREL LEAF	Fear of failure Self-sabotage Self-doubt	Triumphant Perseverance Capable
LAVENDER	Blocked communication Hiding Constricted	Expressive Open Calm
LEMON	Unfocused Fatigued Difficulty learning	Focused Energized Alert
LEMONGRASS	Despairing Hoarding Lethargic	Clarity Simplicity Cleansing
LEMON EUCALYPTUS	Exposed Unprotected Enmeshed	Self-contained Reinforced Protected
LEMON MYRTLE	Mental Fog Confused Negatively influenced	Clarity Rational Intentional
LIME	Disinterested Despairing Resigned Apathetic	Engaged Courageous Determined Grateful

EMOTIONS

ESSENTIAL OIL	NEGATIVE EMOTIONS	POSITIVE PROPERTIES
LITSEA	Limited Stifled Blocked	Manifesting Inspired Aligned
MAGNOLIA	Disconnected Numb Withdrawn Justifying	Connected Compassionate Unified Perceptive
MANUKA	Abandoned Wounded Unsafe	Upheld Comforted Shielded
MARJORAM	Isolated Fear of rejection Cold Distrust	Connected Warm Loving
MELISSA	Burdened Misaligned Darkness	Joyful Integrity Enlightened
MYRRH	Distrusting Ungrounded Unsafe in the world	Safe Secure Trusting Nurtured
NEROLI	Unfulfilled Resentful Aloof	Committed Kind Intimate
NIAOULI	Defensive Irritated Judgmental	Patient Rational Clear Humble
OREGANO	Prideful Willful Opinionated Controlling	Humble Willing Nonattachment Flexible
PATCHOULI	Obsessive Disconnected Body shame	Moderation Balanced Body connection
PEPPERMINT	Heavyhearted Pessimistic Dejected	Buoyant Optimistic Relieved

ESSENTIAL OIL	NEGATIVE EMOTIONS	POSITIVE PROPERTIES
PETITGRAIN	Inherited limitations Dishonoring Unhealthy traditions	Chain-breaking Pioneering Healthy family connections
PINK PEPPER	Self-comparison Self-judgment Judgmental	Equality Self-acceptance Compassionate
RED MANDARIN	Burdened parenting Exhausted Unappreciated	Fulfilled parenting Refreshed Cherished
ROMAN CHAMOMILE	Purposeless Directionless Unsettled	Purposeful Guided Peaceful
ROSE	Unloved Wounded Disheartened	Loved Compassionate Healing
ROSEMARY	Confused Ignorant Uncertain	Mental clarity Knowledgeable Teachable
SANDALWOOD	Prideful Materialistic Distracted	Humble Devotion Spiritual
SIBERIAN FIR	Regretful Loss Fretting	Perspective Wisdom Adapting
SPEARMINT	Inarticulate Timid Withholding voice	Clarity Confident Articulate
SPIKENARD	Ungrateful Victim mentality Resisting	Grateful Acceptance Content
STAR ANISE	Careworn Suppressed Contracted	Regenerated Empowered Expansive

ESSENTIAL OIL	NEGATIVE EMOTIONS	POSITIVE PROPERTIES
TANGERINE	Overburdened Overworked Stifled	Cheerful Spontaneous Creative
TEA TREE	Boundary violation Enmeshed Self-betrayal	Energetic boundaries Respectful connections Resilient
THYME	Unforgiving Intolerant Angry Resentful	Forgiving Tolerant Patient Understanding
TULSI	Misaligned Weakened Blocked	Integrated Healed Harmonized
TURMERIC	Damaged Unsteady Betrayed Oppressed	Resilient Faithful Restored Confident
VETIVER	Scattered Ungrounded Avoiding	Centered Grounded Present
WILD ORANGE	Scarcity Serious Rigid	Abundant Sense of humor Playful
WINTERGREEN	Controlling Self-reliant Willful	Surrender Relying on the Divine Letting go
YARROW | POM	Unsafe Unclear Attacked Energetically weakened	Safe Discerning Protected Strong boundaries
YLANG YLANG	Sadness Joyless Overanalyzing	Freedom Playful Intuitive

OIL BLENDS

ADAPTIV®	Anxious Uneasy Worried	Reassured Calm Clear

EMOTIONS

ESSENTIAL OIL	NEGATIVE EMOTIONS	POSITIVE PROPERTIES
ALIGN	Out of Integrity Imbalanced Distrusting	Aligned Self-acceptance Open
AMĀVĪ®	Resisting male energy Dominant Stressed	Accepting the masculine Integrity Emotional clarity
ANCHOR	Unstable Upheaval Uncertain	Stable Calm Clear
ARISE	Burdened Pessimistic Disconnected	Lifted Enthusiastic Actualized
AROMATOUCH®	Tense Stressed Rigid	Relaxed Balanced Flexible
doTERRA BALANCE®	Ungrounded Disconnected Scattered	Grounded Connected Stable
BEAUTIFUL	Self-critical Abused Grieving Unworthy	Self-respect Healing Lovable Capable
BRAVE®	Afraid Less than Bullied	Courageous Respectful Worthy
doTERRA BREATHE®	Unloved Sad Constricted Grieving	Loved Cared for Receiving Solace
CALMER®	Upset Worried Over-scheduled	Calm Reassured Restful,
doTERRA CHEER®	Pessimistic Burdened Heavyhearted Hopeless	Cheerful Uplifted Hopeful

ESSENTIAL OIL	NEGATIVE EMOTIONS	POSITIVE PROPERTIES
CITRUS BLISS®	Stifled Blocked creativity Unmotivated	Invigorated Creative Motivated
ᵈᵒᵀᴱᴿᴿᴬ CITRUS BLOOM®	Stagnant Immobilized Remorseful	Adventurous Excitement Optimistic
CLARYCALM®	Invulnerable Suffering Guarded	Vulnerable Serene Receptive
ᵈᵒᵀᴱᴿᴿᴬ CONSOLE®	Grieving Loss Traumatized	Comforted Whole Serene
DDR PRIME®	Broken Immobilized Powerless	Repairing Balanced Rebirth Transforming
DEEP BLUE®	Resisting Pained Panicked	Strengthened Soothed Serene
DIGESTZEN®	Unenthusiastic Undernourished Overstimulated	Enthusiastic Nourished Assimilation
ELEVATION	Despairing Discouraged Heavyhearted	Bright Joyful Carefree
ᵈᵒᵀᴱᴿᴿᴬ FORGIVE®	Unforgiving Critical Resentful	Forgiving Understanding Tolerant

ESSENTIAL OIL	NEGATIVE EMOTIONS	POSITIVE PROPERTIES
HARVEST SPICE®	Withdrawn Distracted Blocked	Connected Present Giving
HD CLEAR®	Self-critical Suppressed anger Inadequate	Self-acceptance Worthwhile Ample
HOLIDAY JOY™	Estranged Stressed Cold	Connected Celebratory Warm
HOLIDAY PEACE®	Scattered Unresolved generational issues Ignoring the body's messages	Contemplative Generational healing Restored
dōTERRA HOPE®	Despairing Traumatized Shameful	Hopeful Healing Rebirth
IMMORTELLE	Discouragement Spiritual blindness Spiritually disconnected	Hopeful Transforming Trust in the Divine
INTUNE®	Distracted Procrastinating Overactive	Focused Committed Present
dōTERRA ISLAND MINT®	Overwhelmed Fatigued Heavy	Relaxed Reinvigorated Elevated
dōTERRA MOTIVATE®	Unmotivated Gloomy Weary	Motivated Encouraged Energized
dōTERRA ON GUARD®	Attacked Unprotected Controlled	Protected Capable Independent
dōTERRA PASSION®	Lack of confidence Regimented Joyless	Passionate Risk-taking Spontaneous
PASTTENSE®	Imbalanced Burned out Tense	Equilibrium Calm Relieved

ESSENTIAL OIL	NEGATIVE EMOTIONS	POSITIVE PROPERTIES
dōTERRA PEACE®	Anxious Controlling Attached	Peaceful Content Still
PURIFY	Trapped Negative Toxic	Unencumbered Purifying Clean
RESCUER	Unsettled Chaotic Pained	Soothed Quieted Capable
dōTERRA SERENITY®	Stressed Restless Disconnected	Calm Tranquil Compassionate
SLIM & SASSY®	Worthless Critical Strict	Worthy Acceptance Beautiful
STEADY®	Unstable Incapable Out of control	Steady Grounded Centered
STRONGER®	Weakened Exposed Susceptible	Strengthened Protected Rejuvenated
SUNNY CITRUS	Stagnant Stressed Cynical	Spontaneous Carefree Optimistic
TAMER®	Incongruent Difficulty Assimilating	Integrated Assimilating Clear
TERRASHIELD®	Poor boundaries Attacked Defenseless	Boundaries Safe Self-contained

ESSENTIAL OIL	NEGATIVE EMOTIONS	POSITIVE PROPERTIES
THINKER®	Distracted Inattentive Overstimulated	Focused Attentive Engaged
WHISPER®	Resisting femininity Overly masculine Repressed sexuality	Accepting femininity Soft Healthy sexual expression
ZENDOCRINE®	Dependent Toxic habits Self-sabotage Apathetic	Revitalized Unrestricted Clear

EMOTIONS